Smoking is a

To my old friend Anthony, with best wishes,
Gabriel

July 2017

BY THE SAME AUTHOR

Stop Smoking: Real Help at Last

Smoking is a Psychological Problem

Dr Gabriel Symonds

Why the orthodox approach to smoking cessation is flawed and how you can quit without nicotine, drugs or gimmicks

YOUCAXTON PUBLICATIONS
OXFORD & SHREWSBURY

Copyright © Dr Gabriel Symonds 2016

The Author asserts the moral right to
be identified as the author of this work.

ISBN 978-191117-520-9
Printed and bound in Great Britain.
Published by YouCaxton Publications 2016

All rights reserved. No part of this publication may be reproduced, stored in a retrieval system, or transmitted in any form or by any means, electronic, mechanical, photocopying, recording or otherwise, without the prior permission of the publisher.

This book is sold subject to the condition that it shall not, by way of trade or otherwise, be lent, resold, hired out or otherwise circulated without the publisher's prior consent in any form of binding or cover other than that in which it is published and without a similar condition including this condition being imposed on the subsequent purchaser.

Contents

Introduction 1

PART ONE - SMOKING CESSATION

Chapter 1 - Visions, Stakeholders and Toolkits. 9
Chapter 2 - Stopping Smoking with the NHS. 13
Chapter 3 - Peddling Poison to Doctors 21
Chapter 4 - Smoking in Hospitals 24
Chapter 5 - Banning Smoking in Mental Hospitals 27
Chapter 6 - Smoking in Pregnancy. 31
Chapter 7 - Can't Stop? Won't Stop! 34
Chapter 8 - Cutting Down Forever. 37
Chapter 9 - Mutiny in the Ranks 41
Chapter 10 - Banning Cigarettes 46
Chapter 11 - World Expert on Smoking and Addiction 50
Chapter 12 - What About Allen Carr? 57

PART TWO - HARM REDUCTION

Chapter 13 - Smoking Harm Reduction – a Flawed Concept 63
Chapter 14 - Harm Reduction and the Emperor's New Clothes . . 66
Chapter 15 - Condemning People to Death 72
Chapter 16 - E-Cigarette Circus 77
Chapter 17 - Highly Esteemed Organ 86
Chapter 18 - Waterpipes in Wonderland 90
Chapter 19 - Cigars Are OK – Or Are They? 93
Chapter 20 - Plain Packaging 95

PART THREE - RESEARCH

Chapter 21 - Smoking Research 105
Chapter 22 - Futile Smoking Research 110
Chapter 23 - The Road to Hell 114

PART FOUR - BIG TOBACCO

Chapter 24 - Big Tobacco and the BBC 121
Chapter 25 - Into the Lions' Den 126
Chapter 26 - A Bulldog Named Gladys 132

APPENDIX - The Symonds Method 134

Introduction

In October 2015 a law was passed in Britain forbidding smoking in cars when carrying children. Ever alert to opportunities for creating news, the BBC interviewed two women smokers and a police officer about the new law.[1]

One of the women, Lucy Hardcastle, in the typical smoker's husky voice, said she would ignore the law because she couldn't cope without smoking:

> *It's a drug that I'm needing to take to drive. I don't want to smoke. I've tried to give up so many times. I'm at the stage where having a cigarette makes me feel normal. If I don't have a cigarette I feel jittery and nervous, so that's why I do it.*

The unfortunate Ms Hardcastle's complaints epitomise the tragedy of smoking. Why can't she feel normal without a cigarette? Why does she feel jittery and nervous if she doesn't smoke?

Her life must be terrible. She knows that regularly throughout the day, every day, the dreaded jitteriness and nervousness will come upon her if not pre-empted or relieved by another dose of the poison nicotine. How does she get on at night though? Does she wake every hour to have a cigarette? I doubt it.

What she needs to understand is that *these feelings are caused by nicotine withdrawal*. But if she *doesn't* relieve them with another dose of nicotine, what will happen? Will they become intolerable? No. *They will go away*. And never come back – unless she puts more nicotine into her body.

Just reading this, however, is unlikely to do it for her – though it might. Stopping smoking without tears requires full

---

[1] http://www.bbc.co.uk/programmes/p0341lqq

explanation and advice from a knowledgeable and supportive counsellor. The counsellor, moreover, should not recommend any form of nicotine product or drugs. I have successfully treated many patients like Lucy Hardcastle simply by helping them to understand why quitting *seems* so hard and how this can provide the key to easy smoking cessation – to the gratification of both patient and doctor.

How not to cure the smoking epidemic

In this book I aim to show how the current approach of the British and other governments to the smoking problem is wrong-headed. It's based on the idea that the prevalence of smoking can be gradually reduced by what is called tobacco control: strong health warnings and horrible pictures on cigarette packs, standard (plain) packaging, restrictions on where you're allowed to smoke, increased cigarette taxation, etc. These measures assume smokers can be persuaded by logic and while they may have some effect, they don't take account of the fact that *smoking is largely a psychological problem*. In any case, the very phrase 'tobacco control' shows the wrong emphasis. I argue that tobacco doesn't need to be controlled; it needs to be *abolished*.

Further, I try to show why the current conventional approach to smoking cessation is likely to be more of a hindrance than a help for smokers wanting to quit. With prominence given to nicotine products and/or drugs, it reinforces the idea that quitting is difficult. In fact, it seems to be regarded as so difficult that those who promote these methods themselves don't have much confidence in them. One authoritative source (see Chapter 14) provides a cop-out for smokers – assuming such exist – who 'may not be able or do not want to stop smoking, or who want to reduce the amount they smoke, or who want to stop smoking without giving up nicotine'. The solution to their smoking problem? More nicotine. With *licensed* products – gum, patches, e-cigarettes, etc.

Introduction

What's wrong with so-called nicotine replacement therapy (NRT)?
If you're a smoker seeking professional help to quit, there's almost a knee-jerk response to provide you with NRT. I believe such an approach is wrong.
Here's why:

- The name is misleading. It means neither that nicotine is the replacement of something nor that nicotine is to be replaced with something. It really means nicotine *maintenance* therapy. NRT merely allows smokers to continue taking the poison nicotine into their bodies in a way other than by smoking cigarettes, and so it *keeps the addiction going*.
- NRT reinforces the mistaken idea that stopping smoking is terribly difficult without medical help.
- NRT makes smokers reliant on some outside agency to assist in the task of quitting, implying they're unable to do it unaided. It thus disempowers and even infantilises smokers.
- If a smoker tries NRT and fails to stop smoking, there's an inbuilt excuse: *it* didn't work!
- Even if it does work, when you tear off the last patch or spit out the last piece of gum, what's to stop you from starting smoking again?
- This approach to smoking cessation implies it's mainly or entirely a physical problem, so if only you can get over the awful withdrawal symptoms and cravings, you'll never want to smoke again.
- The recommendation to use NRT does little or nothing to help the smoker understand why he or she smokes in the first place and why it *seems* so difficult to quit. This understanding can empower smokers to stop easily and permanently.

Similar considerations apply to prescription drugs (bupropion or varenicline) used in smoking cessation.

Hoist with their own petards

As in my first book, I make extensive use of quotations from the literature on smoking, including papers in scholarly journals, official reports and other publications. This curious branch of literature is critically discussed, and I make no apology for straying into satire which so much of it invites. In their own words, the authors often demonstrate (as well as their all-too-common poor use of English which sometimes degenerates into incomprehensibility and even illiteracy) how the research they do seems designed either to prove the obvious or merely to produce more papers to add to the already voluminous literature on smoking and to look good on the authors' CVs. The practical application of this ever-growing pile of papers is often left unstated, or the authors merely conclude that more research is needed.

Overview of this book

Part I examines the smoking cessation methods promulgated by the NHS and attempts to show how nearly all are inherently discouraging to would-be quitters. They emphasise the difficulties smokers will face, that they will need will power and it will take a long time. Worse, a list of unpleasant withdrawal symptoms is usually mentioned and to cope with these some form of nicotine treatment or a prescription drug is recommended. In my view this is based on flawed research and fails to take into account the true nature of smoking.

Part II looks at the 'harm reduction' approach to the smoking epidemic, and explains why this is also a flawed concept. Harm reduction means that smokers who wish to keep using nicotine for its illusory benefits should be encouraged, in effect, to continue to be addicted to this poison in a supposedly safer way. I argue this is unnecessary, defeatist and likely to result in millions of people using nicotine long-term, especially by e-cigarettes, as is already happening. Satirical critiques of waterpipes, cigars and the flawed science behind the push for plain (standard) packaging are also included.

Part III deals with some aspects of smoking research. It is evident that the authors of many published papers see publication as an end in itself, often getting side-tracked into academic backwaters of little or no practical relevance. Are there racial differences in smokers? (And if there are, what do we do about it?) Do we really need brain scans to help people stop smoking? Is there any point in investigating such questions as whether 'health warnings on cigarette packs are consistent prospective predictors of making quit attempts'? (Chapter 23.)

In *Part IV* the question is raised by implication whether, in terms of the numbers of deaths caused by smoking, there is similarity between the activities of Big Tobacco and the Holocaust.

The *Appendix* contains a condensed version of the Symonds Method of smoking cessation which is set out in full in my previous book: *Stop Smoking: Real Help at Last*.

New approach needed

The whole approach to smoking cessation needs to change. The emphasis should shift away from NRT, e-cigarettes and drugs to being nicotine- and drug-free. More attention should be paid to evidence (see Chapter 9) which shows the best way to stop smoking is – just stop. With the right kind of counselling this is can be very easy to do, in my experience.

Secondly, the stress on unpleasant withdrawal symptoms should cease. These are merely lists that get copied from one article or internet source to another as if they are gospel truths. Instead of *telling* people all the awful things they are likely to experience, they should be asked open-ended questions:

'What, if anything, do you feel when you feel like having a cigarette?' The answers – or often, the lack of an answer – may be surprising. The reality is that for most people the withdrawal symptoms are *not that bad*. There may be some discomfort, but it's by no means unbearable. Unfortunately, people *believe* it will be terrible because this is what they're told: if you expect you'll go through hell that's likely what you'll feel, so quitting smoking will be a struggle.

Thirdly, the government needs to enact legislation with a realistic and short timetable – say no more than five years – to disestablish tobacco companies and ban the sale of tobacco products. It must be made clear to the public that smoking is legalised drug addiction which kills 100,000 people a year in Britain – an unacceptable situation.

A word on nomenclature

Some years ago there was a suggestion by a human rights organization that states ruled by regimes that routinely torture their opponents should be referred to as 'the torture state of …', for example, 'the torture state of North Korea'. In the same way I think that whenever nicotine is mentioned it should be prefixed by the word 'poison', which is how it is referred to in this book (allowing for context).

Secondly, in discussions about the smoking problem, the phrase 'tobacco control', with the related expressions 'tobacco-control community' and even 'health community', regularly crop up. In this context the idea of community seems merely to refer to individuals working independently in the fields of tobacco research and smoking cessation. The main outcome of so much of this activity is the production of scientific papers, much of it to dubious effect. For reasons explained in Chapter 21, I shall refer to this so-called community by what I consider a more appropriate term: the Tobacco-Control Industry.

PART ONE
Smoking Cessation

Chapter 1

Visions, Stakeholders and Toolkits

Typical of the great effort that the NHS is putting in to 'control' tobacco is the publication of a booklet called *Tobacco Control Alliances: a Toolkit for London*.[2] Written by one Ms Leona Condliffe on behalf of the London Regional Tobacco Policy Team, her main qualification seems to have been her ability to write gobbledegook without blushing. She was assisted in this wheeze by seventeen other people who held positions in their respective organisations such as (don't laugh) Regional Tobacco Policy Manager, Assistant Regional Tobacco Policy Manager, Senior Tobacco Policy Manager, Tobacco Control National Support Team Delivery Manger, Tobacco Control National Support Team Associate Delivery Manager, Tobacco Control Alliance Co-ordinator, etc.

The style of writing I don't think would win any prizes in the Plain English Campaign:

> *To create the vision for the Alliance, it is essential that partners are brought together to share ideas and values and to build connections with each other.*
>
> *When people connect with each other, they build trust, and when they build trust they are able to create synergy.*

Vision in this context I suppose means a vivid concept or mental picture; synergy means working together.

Why such a cumbersome way of putting it? The word

---

[2] www.google.com/search?q=tobacco+control+alliances+a+toolkit+for+long on&ie=utf-8&oe=utf-8#q=tobacco+control+alliances+a+toolkit+for+london

vision doesn't sit comfortably here, nor does the concept of creating synergy.

Why not simply say, 'To develop the Alliance, ideas need be shared.'

But it's hardly necessary to say even this as it's stating the obvious.

One could take almost any passage at random from this splendid publication to find a candidate for inclusion in *Pseuds' Corner* in *Private Eye*.[3] For example:

> *The comprehensive tobacco control agenda requires a structure that supports clear accountability and strategic decision-making as well as allowing for a wide range of partners with different fields of expertise and interests to engage at different levels…[The] suggested structure for the governance and coordination of tobacco control…is essentially made up of a core group of partners, who meet regularly to take a strategic overview and co-ordinate delivery across key delivery streams. The implementation of these delivery streams is addressed through a number of operational groups…and it may not be necessary to address each delivery stream in a separate group.*

Or how about this passage with repetitive use of the wretched word 'stakeholder'. Couldn't she have used a word like 'participant' or a phrase such as 'interested party'?

> *A stakeholder is any individual, organisation or group who may be either positively or negatively affected by the work of the partnership.*
>
> *Once you have identified your local stakeholders, conducting a stakeholder analysis will help you to map local stakeholders*

---

[3] The British satirical magazine.

Visions, Stakeholders and Toolkits

in terms of their interest in and influence over the Alliance, and to identify the different levels at which you will need to engage people. Figure 2 is a basic stakeholder analysis matrix to help you to do this.

In one of the appendixes she really goes to town over stakeholders, not to mention keys and levers for engagement. (Layout paraphrased.)

> *This section will cover: Key Local Authority tobacco control stakeholders and levers for engagement. Key NHS tobacco control stakeholders and levers for engagement. Wider stakeholders and levers for engagement.*
> *Appendix 6.1: Key stakeholders and priorities. This section provides an overview of key tobacco control stakeholders and levers to engage them in local tobacco control work. This stakeholder analysis is by no means exhaustive, and there will be other people in your Borough who could contribute to both the Alliance and local work programmes. This section is presented in three main sections: 1. a) Key Local Authority stakeholders b) Key levers to engage with Local Authority stakeholders 2. a) Key NHS stakeholders b) Key levers to engage NHS stakeholders 3. Wider stakeholders Appendix g.1.1 Local Authority Stakeholders...*

Then we have:

> *The Tobacco Control Alliance Lead should ideally be a dedicated post working at a senior level to provide strategic leadership to partnership development and the delivery of tobacco control work programmes...*

And this:

Smoking is a Psychological Problem

Stopping the inflow of young people recruited as smokers.

You don't need inflow and recruited in the same sentence. How about simply 'Stopping young people becoming smokers'. Apart from all the key levers to engage local authority stakeholders and delivery of tobacco control interventions (groan), I would take her up on one point. Ms Condliffe wants, rightly, to abolish smoking in schools, but this is what she says:

> *The development of a No Smoking Policy for the school is a criterion for Healthy Schools and is recommended by NICE. The smokefree policy should meet the following criteria: The school is a smokefree site (**with the exception of the caretaker's house**)...* (Emphasis added.)

Why is the caretaker's house the patronizing exception in a non-smoking school?

Chapter 2

Stopping Smoking with the NHS

Smokefree campaign

Let's look at the help offered to people who want to stop smoking by the British National Health Service (NHS).

They have what they call a Smokefree Campaign which is available as a web-based or mobile phone app. If you sign up you get sent for the next twenty-eight days motivational messages and encouragement.

Although presented in a cheerful upbeat style, with a background of blue sky, sun, trees, flowers and stick figures with their arms raised in exultation, the Campaign inadvertently reinforces the difficulties and temptations the anonymous copywriters think would-be quitters will have to deal with.

You're also told that you're up to four times more likely to stay Smokefree with so-called stop-smoking medicines and face-to-face support. What this really means, however, is that without help only 4% stop but with help 15% stop. So, of one hundred smokers who accept such assistance, a year later eighty-five are still smoking.

Also, the frequent references to stop-smoking medicines, that is, nicotine products and drugs, imply that you will need this kind of help. To obtain these you are advised to consult, not just your friendly neighbourhood pharmacist, but your pharmacy team, or your GP or local Stop-Smoking Service.

The campaign offers simplistic advice to help you endure the suffering you are likely to experience after stopping smoking. If you get through the first five days, 'It might have seemed the longest five days ever' and 'To help you cope, keep yourself busy until the craving passes, or try these: going for a walk, playing a game on your mobile or computer, or phoning a friend.'

If this doesn't work, to beat those awful withdrawal symptoms, stop-smoking medicines are the way to go!

> *Talk to your pharmacy team, GP or local Stop Smoking Service about stop smoking medicines that can help with nicotine withdrawal symptoms.*
>
> *When you stop smoking, you can experience nicotine withdrawal symptoms such as cravings, headaches, feeling irritable and having trouble sleeping. Stop smoking medicines can reduce these symptoms and help you stop for good.*
>
> *If you're using stop smoking medicine, make sure you've got enough to keep you going for the next seven days.*
>
> *Stop smoking medicines can help if you're feeling irritable. Already using them and still feeling grumpy? This could be a sign you're not using them correctly, so check with your GP or pharmacist.*
>
> *Remember stop smoking medicines can help you manage your cravings.*
>
> *A common mistake people can make is to stop using their product too soon. This includes both nicotine replacement therapy (NRT) and Champix (varenicline).* ***It is easy to mistake a lack of discomfort for a belief that the addiction to nicotine is over. Treatment normally lasts for 12 weeks and stopping early can mean cravings return.*** *The best option is to speak to a pharmacist, local stop smoking adviser or your GP.* (Emphasis added.)

In my view this is seriously misleading and arbitrary. How is one to tell that the addiction is over if not by the absence of discomfort? Are you supposed to have discomfort unless it's suppressed by drugs? And why should treatment last for twelve weeks? Why not thirteen or seven-and-a-half weeks? It is well known the 'cravings' can recur periodically even for years after finishing conventional smoking cessation treatment. And if you do stop with the dubious assistance of stop-smoking medicine, what's to prevent you starting smoking again?

Now, what about these stop-smoking medicines?

If you're one of the unfortunate smokers for whom 'nicotine cravings [are] the hardest thing to handle' one of the ways to deal with this, it seems, is to keep putting nicotine into your body but by a different route. To wit: using nicotine gum, patches, lozenges, 'inhalators' or 'microtabs'. Here are a few illustrative quotes from what they say about some of these:

> *Gum: When you quit you should be chewing about one piece of gum every hour...chew until the taste becomes strong or hot. After this you can rest the gum inside your cheek... gradually you can cut down on the amount of gum you use... some people dislike the taste...*
>
> *Patches: They work by releasing nicotine directly into the bloodstream through the skin...the 24-hour patch may cause some sleep disturbance but is helpful for people who have strong cravings during the early morning.*
>
> *Inhalators: A nicotine inhalator works by releasing nicotine vapour when you suck on it...you should use yours whenever you feel strong cravings for a cigarette...You should aim to use the inhalator for a total of 12 weeks...Use from 6 to 12 cartridges a day for the first eight weeks...when you experience cravings for a cigarette.*
>
> *Nasal spray: [Apply] one spray into each nostril twice an hour...for a total of 12 weeks. The nicotine nasal spray is the strongest form of nicotine replacement therapy. This can be a very useful and effective form of medication for highly dependent heavy smokers who have difficulty giving up using other methods...[It]may cause side effects such as nose and throat irritation, coughing, and watering eyes.*

Not very inviting, is it.

Other stop-smoking medicines, i.e., drugs
What if these various nicotine products don't work? Then you can turn to the other type of stop-smoking medicines. Except they aren't. Nonetheless, two prescription drugs are in use as smoking cessation aids, though Smokefree only mentions varenicline (Champix); the other is known as bupropion (Zyban, Wellbutrin). Varenicline is a selective nicotine-receptor partial agonist. Bupropion's main use is as an antidepressant, and although the way it works isn't fully understood it's thought to be dopaminergic and/or noradrenergic. (This means it's believed to have effects on two different types of brain cells.) Both drugs have a list of possible side-effects as long as your arm. Some of the more important are, for bupropion: suicidal thoughts and behaviour especially in young people, palpitations, headache, agitation, dizziness and insomnia; and for varenicline: headache, suicidal ideas, sleep disorders, chest pain in 4% of users and 1% may suffer heart attacks.

Stoptober
There is also a stop-smoking scheme offered by NHS England called Stoptober, presumably because it was launched in the month of October, in 2014.

Like the Smokefree campaign it's the conventional approach with the usual built-in discouragement. They seem to recognise this fact and try to make a joke of it:

> *Welcome to Day 1 of Stoptober. Now, it's fair to say that this is the toughest day. Why? Because people keep coming up to you telling you it's the toughest day.*
> *Day 2. You may also feel a bit dizzy… carbon monoxide has disappeared from your body and your lungs will start to clear of* (sic) *mucus and other toxins.* [I didn't know mucus was a toxin.]

> *Day 3. GRRRRRRRR!!!! (sic)... If you are feeling a bit emotional or moody, don't worry that's normal and it will get easier. Tell your friends and family that you might be a little snappy for a couple of days.*

Inevitably, there's dumbed-down vulgarity:

> *Day 4. Just think, on your next night out, you can get ejected from a nightclub, spill a kebab down your top, get told to p*** off by an attractive member of the opposite sex and - if you haven't smoked - it's still a triumph!*

Back to Day 3. Linking to Facebook reveals an appeal from a desperate sounding woman:

> *wish u had more info on here as to the different things that stopping smoking can make u feel, ie , spaced out lack of concentration, which isn't good when ur driving, just nodding off, lack of sleep at night, constant urge for loo, xtra peeing, achy eatling more , bloating , wind, . it would help more people if these subjects were covered on this official site , its not always about the craving, I want to understand whats going on with my body and why its affected in this way, it is that what keeps my incentive up, but would love more info*

She's on the right lines (even if her punctuation is wobbly) since nobody *does* explain it to her. It seems these unpleasant feelings are regarded as a normal and inevitable part of stopping smoking and the best that can be done is to support quitters through this difficult time by motivational sound bites. I sympathize with this woman and the many others who use social media to air their problems. Fortunately, however, all this is nonsense. There's no need to go through such suffering.

With a positive attitude and if you're helped to understand what happens when you stop poisoning yourself with nicotine, in practice you're likely to experience very little difficulty. And you won't need stop-smoking medicines.

What happens if you attend a free NHS local Stop-Smoking Service? It's more of the same:

> *You will find trained advisers on hand to support you, either one-to-one or in a group…Your adviser will be able to tell you about nicotine replacement products and other stop smoking medicines. They can also recommend which product or combination of products could work for you…Your adviser can measure the levels of carbon monoxide in your body (the CO level) using a carbon monoxide monitor…*[4]

Do you really need a read-out on a monitor to be convinced you're poisoning yourself by smoking and does this knowledge make it easier to quit?

Stoptober – 2015 version

A new edition was put out in October 2015. When I signed up for it for research purposes I received a message:

> *Support, fun, games and exclusive content from our comedians to get you through the 28 days in our app.*

It sounds like they're trying to make stopping smoking a joke, with fun and games to get through the next twenty-eight days. And then what? How are you going to get through the rest of your life?

More introductory information:

---

[4] http://www.nhs.uk/smokefree/help-and-advice/local-support-services-helplines

> This year we've got loads of extra support from some funny new friends. Rhod Gilbert will be sending you messages with some tough love, and words of comfort will come from Shappi Khorsandi. Bill Bailey will be providing some distractions to keep your mind off things and Al Murray will be there with some good old fashioned common sense.

Except for the bit about common sense this nicely sums up what's wrong with the current standard approach to smoking cessation: you need loads of support, tough love, comfort and distractions.

The day before the series started I got a one minute video featuring the cheerful cockney comedian, Al Murray, which was actually quite amusing: smoking cessation through humour!

Each day you're sent another short video, as follows:

Day 1. Stopping smoking for 28 days is likened to climbing 28 molehills rather than mountains but, we're warned, it's 'no walk in the park'.

Day 2. 'So you made it to day two already. Excellent!' Then, 'some ideas to keep your minds and hands busy.' Such as: cut an orange into several pieces which you can put back together again like a puzzle, wood carving or making a scale model of a road junction with old shoe-laces.

Day 3. This video shows the comedienne Shappi Khorsandi trying to relax in a bubble bath, 'because Day 3 can be tough.'

Day 4. To take your mind off cigarettes it's suggested you stick a picture of something you don't like, such as yourself or some cigarettes, onto a cushion and you then bash this with your fist till you feel better. Quite funny in a way.

Day 5. '…I know you might be feeling a bit restless, so here's a quick idea for keeping you distracted…take up train spotting.'

Day 6. The video features more encouragement from the cockney comedian – quite amusing.

Day 7. 'Well done! You made it through seven days. That's brilliant!' To celebrate, funny man Bill Bailey puts an enormous candle on a lentil and nettle cake. So ridiculous it's quite amusing. What's not amusing is the accompanying message: 'If you're using stop smoking medicines, remember to stock up for the next seven days. Good luck!'

If I was a still smoker I'd rather eat lentil and nettle cake which 'hits the spot every time' than dull my brain with another drug to get off the drug nicotine.

Day 8. You're reminded of the money you save by not smoking.

Day 9. While playing the piano one these characters tells you that your sleep patterns by now should be returning to normal, implying that you would have had difficulty sleeping as a result of stopping smoking. A bit more piano playing and – that's it!

Day 10. Now we have lavatorial humour, inevitably.

Day 11. A party trick is shown of putting some coins on your elbow and with a quick movement catching them in your hand.

At this point I decided I'd seen enough.

Chapter 3

Peddling Poison to Doctors

How are nicotine products promoted to doctors? Some recent issues of the scholarly journal that styles itself *Tobacco Control* carry full-page colour advertisements for a product called Nicorette, a nicotine-containing skin patch.[5] Common side effects are listed in small print: headache, dizziness, nausea, vomiting, GI (stomach) discomfort and erythema (redness of the skin). Don't know if I like the sound of that. Anyway, one advertisement features a model called Ryan who, it says, is 'doing something incredible' and 'he's also running his fastest 10K ever.' Is he, indeed? (I presume by K they mean km.) Although it's likely a smoker will be able to run faster if he stops smoking, it stretches one's credulity that a smoker could run 10km even slowly, or would try to.[6]

The punch line is that people like Ryan with your 'continuous support' (whatever that means) and drug treatment such as Nicorette are 'nearly four times more likely to quit smoking for good than those offered no support.' But the sentence ends with the underwhelming qualification that this is only 15% v. 4%, as noted in the previous chapter.

The advertisement says the patches should be used daily for eight weeks (not twelve weeks as advised by the NHS Smokefree campaign) after which 'gradual weaning from the patch should be initiated.' Sounds like this will do a power of good – for the manufacturer.

---

[5] For example, November 2014 and March 2015.

[6] This could almost come from a Ken Dodd-type joke. A doctor comes to see a patient who has had surgery to his hands. 'Doctor,' says the man excitedly, holding up his bandaged hands, 'Will I be able to play the piano when these bandages come off?' 'I don't see why not.' replies the doctor. 'That's wonderful,' says the patient, 'I couldn't play it before.'

Smoking is a Psychological Problem

On opening the cover of the November 2015 edition of the aforementioned august organ, I was confronted by what at first glance looked like an ad for a packet of washing powder. Closer inspection, however, revealed it was an illiterate puff for 'extra strength gum for enhanced craving relief', which turned out to be the same Nicorette chewing gum but containing 6mg of the poison nicotine instead of the usual 2mg or 4mg.

Not quite sure about the 'enhanced craving relief'. Do they perhaps mean enhanced relief of craving? They claim it's 'for smokers of more than twenty cigarettes a day.' So if you smoke twenty-one or more cigarettes a day you'll either suffer enhanced cravings or you'll need enhanced relief from your cravings, it seems. Anyway, the new strength fruit flavoured nicotine gum, they say, 'is indicated to aid smokers wishing to quit.'

Hold it right there! The word 'indicate' in medical parlance means a desirable or necessary course of action. Who says if you want to stop smoking, that is, get rid of nicotine, it's desirable or necessary to use nicotine? Even the makers of this product seem to have doubts about it because if you read the small print carefully it says: 'It is indicated…to assist smokers who are unable or unwilling to smoke.' (The same wording appears in the ad featuring our friend Ryan, above.)

This is actually what is says. Well, if you're a smoker who's unable or unwilling to smoke, the problem's solved, right?

Let's plough on through the small print. We have: 'If the patient smokes twenty cigarettes or less (*sic*) per day, 2mg nicotine gum is indicated.' Pity they can't write proper English. But it's just as well to stick with lower doses, assuming anyone needs the poison nicotine at all, because some people who have quit smoking with the hindrance of nicotine gum have difficulty discontinuing the gum. What should they do? The advertiser has the answer: 'Contact their doctor or pharmacist for advice.' Under these circumstances, I wonder what else would such unfortunate people contact their doctor or pharmacist for, if not advice.

Talking of advice, they do inform you that: 'After about 30 minutes of [use] the gum will be exhausted.' And so, presumably, will the user.

By the way, the reference to back up the claim that this new extra-strength nicotine gum is indicated for smokers of more than twenty cigarettes a day, is to a conference poster presentation written by three people who all are employees of, er, the company that makes the gum!

Chapter 4

Smoking in Hospitals

What to do about smoking in hospitals? The National Institute for Health and Care Excellence (NICE), in a paper entitled *Smoking: acute, maternity and mental health services*, enlightens us.[7]
They set out their aims:

> This guidance aims to support smoking cessation, temporary abstinence from smoking and smokefree policies in all secondary care (hospital) settings.

A couple of links later we come to the nitty-gritty:

> Stop smoking services provide a combination of behavioural support and pharmacotherapy to aid smoking cessation.

If we delve a little further, behavioural support aggrandizes into 'Intensive behavioural support'. And what does that consist of?

Well, intensive behavioural support, we are told, involves 'meetings between someone who smokes...and a counsellor trained to provided stop smoking support.' (Sigh.) And then what happens?

> The discussions may include information, practical advice about goal-setting, self-monitoring and dealing with the barriers to stopping smoking as well as encouragement.

---

[7] http://www.nice.org.uk/guidance/ph48

> *Intensive behavioural support also includes anticipating and dealing with the challenges of stopping...Established and effective behaviour-change techniques should be used...*

Having to wade through all this goal-setting, self-monitoring, barriers to stopping, challenges of stopping, behaviour-change techniques, etc., is enough to make a smoker want a cigarette!

Why make it so complicated? The goal and the behavioural change are the same: stop smoking. It seems to me that some of the challenges and barriers to quitting are those put up by this kind of so-called intensive support.

It gets worse:

> *Support is typically offered weekly for at least the first 4 weeks of a quit attempt...and [is] normally given with stop smoking pharmacotherapy (prescription drugs).*

Note it's only a quit attempt (as if the counsellor half-expects the smoker to fail), the process goes on for at least four weeks and drugs are used as well.

This is just the preamble. If we click on 'Go straight to the recommendations' we find a list of seventeen of these.

Here goes:

> *Recommendation 1. Develop a local behaviour change policy and strategy.*

This leads to:

- *Ensure policies and strategies aim to improve everyone's health and wellbeing*
- *Use health equity audit to ensure health inequalities will not increase, and if possible will decrease as a result of the*

> *local behaviour change strategy and related programmes and interventions...*
> - *Develop a commissioning strategy, linked to relevant policies, for an evidence-based behaviour change programme of population, community, organisational and individual-level behaviour change interventions...*
> - *Work with the local community to develop the strategy...*

The reader will forgive me if I stop here, because I'm falling asleep.

No matter how much you exercise your left-click finger, nowhere could I find any indication of what you are actually supposed to do to change someone's behaviour. One can only marvel at the cost and man-hours which must have gone into creating this meaningless twaddle.

Chapter 5

Banning Smoking in Mental Hospitals

Arguments for and against banning smoking in British mental hospitals are presented in a recent edition of *The British Medical Journal*.[8] This paper exemplifies the lack of understanding of the nature of smoking and the way to deal effectively with it which are to be found in so many papers in the medical literature.

In favour of a ban, Deborah Arnott, chief executive of ASH, points out the many advantages of quitting, including improvement in mental and well as physical heath, and notes that psychiatric patients are as motivated to quit as anyone else. She also indicates two reasons for the high prevalence of smoking among mental inpatients: everyone else is doing it, and there is 'simply nothing else to do.' What a sad indictment of the way these hospitals are run.

With outdoor smoking being exempted from the ban on smoking in public places in the UK, these patients are being indirectly encouraged to keep smoking, with smoking breaks every one or two hours. Ms Arnott makes an interesting further observation about this state of affairs: '…[nicotine] addicted service users (euphemism for mental patients) are forced into withdrawal several times a day…' Does she realise, I wonder, that smokers who are not mental patients are also forced into withdrawal several times a day – by the very nature of smoking?

If mental patients were not allowed to smoke outdoors as well, they would effectively be forced to quit smoking, she says.

---
[8] BMJ 2015;351:h5654

Would this be such a bad thing? The English Court of Appeal doesn't think so since it has declared that smoking cannot be considered a fundamental human right.

It's also mentioned that although some mental-patient smokers don't want to quit because they think cigarettes help reduce stress, in fact '…smoking has no positive effect, and any perceived benefits primarily relate to relief from cravings.' Indeed, but she thinks the way to deal with this, in the fashion of the prestigious Maudsley Hospital, is to offer nicotine maintenance therapies, including e-cigarettes, soon after these patients enter the ward.

Patients admitted to mental hospitals by definition are in a state of distress and will usually be given tranquillisers and other drugs to calm them down. This should deal with the temporary additional anxiety which people stopping smoking may experience from nicotine withdrawal.

As I have said before, offering nicotine as a 'treatment' for smoking merely perpetuates the idea that it's terribly hard to stop without medical help, and keeps the addiction going.

In my view, mental-hospital staff should teach smokers that smoking actually increases anxiety through nicotine withdrawal, but after a few days of not smoking they won't experience this additional source of anxiety any more. Medicinal nicotine, therefore, is not only unnecessary but counterproductive.

There's no need for mental patients to be treated differently from anyone else with respect to their smoking. And if they feel driven to smoke out of boredom, surely part of the treatment should be the provision of meaningful occupation of some sort.

Ms Arnott ends by saying, 'We should no longer condone patients smoking themselves to death while in our care.' Quite right.

On the other side of the debate, Michael Fitzpatrick, a former GP, thinks 'Blanket smoking bans…prevent [patients] from taking responsibility for their own actions' and that 'exercise of their independent will [to smoke] is important to recovery.'

He further asserts that:

> Depriving psychiatric patients of their autonomy – their right to make choices relating to their health – means treating them like children...Many people with mental illness think they derive pleasure from smoking and enjoy smoking with others; if deprived of cigarettes they may become irritable.

Note the reiteration of the notion of deprivation, with the resultant dispossession of the right to make choices and the irritability from not smoking.

Smoking, once you start, isn't a choice; it's a compulsion due to nicotine addiction. Further, the irritability smokers may experience shortly after the last cigarette is something they suffer from all their smoking lives. He implies that this is due to a smoker being deprived of pleasure and enjoyment, but as will readily become apparent if one takes the trouble to talk with smokers, smoking is not inherently pleasurable or enjoyable. These are illusions due to relief of the temporary displeasure and irritability caused by nicotine withdrawal.

For smoking cessation to be successful, therefore, it's important that smokers are helped to understand that if they quit they're not being deprived of anything. On the contrary, they will probably feel *much better* because they will no longer suffer repeated withdrawal symptoms.

Dr Fitzpatrick's worry seems to be that a blanket prohibition will leave patients feeling resentful and likely to relapse to smoking on leaving hospital. On the contrary, I would argue that it's patronizing and demeaning for smokers in mental hospitals to be treated in such a way as to imply they're so feeble they can't manage without smoking and that they should immediately be offered nicotine-maintenance therapy.

These days, if you go into a café in Britain you will, in all likelihood, find a prominent notice saying, 'It is against the law to smoke in these premises.' Does this make a smoker popping in for a cuppa and a plate of egg and chips feel deprived? Does a smoker on a long distance flight feel deprived and resentful that smoking is prohibited on board the aircraft?

While the good doctor admonishes that 'Psychiatric health workers should concentrate their energies on the treatment of mental illness…' his answer to patients complaining of '…lack of purposeful activity in overcrowded and understaffed wards, and of…boredom, frustration, and inactivity...' is that some respite is provided by smoking breaks. What he doesn't seem to understand is that mental patients' symptoms are likely made worse by their smoking and will be improved by quitting.[9] Therefore, smoking cessation, voluntary or enforced by legislation, should be considered an important part of the treatment.

---

[9] BMJ 2014;348:g1151

Chapter 6

Smoking in Pregnancy

For an update on the official stance on the serious problem of smoking by pregnant women, there's an editorial in *The British Medical Journal* written by a woman who is a lecturer in addictions at the UK Centre for Tobacco and Alcohol Studies.[10] So she should know what she's talking about.

First, we're reminded of the unfortunate fact that in England 12% of pregnant women smoke through to delivery. Then the obvious is underlined:

> In addition to the countless negative consequences for the smoker's own mental and physical health, smoking in pregnancy is linked to a wide range of poor health outcomes for the child. Thus there is an urgent need to help pregnant smokers who find it difficult to quit [but] a randomised placebo controlled trial found no benefit of transdermal nicotine patches in pregnant smokers' smoking abstinence.

As for drugs used smoking cessation:

> ...evidence on the effectiveness and efficacy of drug treatments for pregnant smokers is lacking... and cannot be recommended.

So much for that.

However, on an upbeat note she says:

> ...good evidence shows that psychosocial interventions help pregnant smokers to quit.

---

[10] BMJ 2014;348:g1808

By psychosocial interventions she means:

> Individual counselling, financial incentives, peer support, and feedback on fetal health or the by-products of tobacco smoking (for example, measuring the levels of carbon monoxide in expired air).

But then we're back at square one:

> ...practitioners supporting pregnant smokers...should routinely intervene [by] offering help and advice [and this] should be followed by referral to specialist smoking cessation services or instigation of other intensive and evidence based behavioural support.

And the practical conclusion of all this?

> ...it may be too early to abandon the option of nicotine replacement therapy (NRT) entirely...a much greater effort is still needed to identify, test, and deliver more effective treatments for pregnant smokers who struggle to quit.

It seems NRT is no good, so try psychosocial interventions, peer support and financial rewards.

The coy term financial rewards, otherwise known as bribery, is also discussed in another editorial in *The British Medical Journal*.[11] Here, the absurdity, even desperation, of this way of trying to stop pregnant women harming themselves and their unborn babies through smoking is reflected in the result of a quoted trial:

> ...it remains disappointing that 77% of pregnant smokers failed to quit despite the offer of £400 in shopping vouchers.

---
[11] BMJ 2015;350:h297

The average cost of a pack of cigarettes in the UK in 2014 was £8.47. If a pack-a-day woman stopped smoking for the forty weeks of her pregnancy, apart from gaining great health benefits, she would avoid wasting £2,372. Would it make a difference if they offered a more realistic bribe, say £3,000? (The researchers found that they needed to offer bribes to 7.2 pregnant smokers to get one to stop, so the cost per 'success' was £2,880.)

The editorial also reminds us:

> *Cigarette dependence is both physiological and psychological, and cessation techniques include counselling, cognitive and behavioural therapy, hypnosis, acupuncture, and drug treatment.*

Here the lack of understanding of why people smoke and why they apparently find it so difficult to stop is evident. Yes, cigarette (nicotine) dependence is both physiological (physical) and psychological, but what is not generally realised is that it's about 90% psychological and only about 10% physical, in my experience. Cessation techniques may well include counselling, but what sort of counselling? Offering cognitive and behavioural therapy, hypnosis, acupuncture, drugs and what have you not, merely reflect the bankruptcy of the current approach to smoking cessation: none of these methods is much good.

Chapter 7

Can't Stop? Won't Stop!

The mental side-effects the drug varenicline mentioned in Chapter 2, particularly depression and suicidal thoughts, are discussed in another editorial in *The British Medical Journal*[12], so this is something doctors should take very seriously.

One phrase caught my eye: 'patients struggling to stop smoking'

The idea of struggling to do something, such as losing weight, is perfectly understandable, and there is no easy answer for many people who have a weight problem.

However, in regard to smoking this is a rather curious way of putting it. It suggests either that these smokers wish to stop but can't overcome a compulsion to keep smoking, or that they don't want to stop but struggle against this with their knowledge of the health hazards. Or maybe it's both.

The dilemma is well put by the actor Jeremy Irons in a 1987 video:

> *For two days I tried to stop. I didn't tell anybody. I didn't tell my wife. And I became intolerable. I actually became a creature from another planet, a creature from the Blue Lagoon…I became a horrendous person, and life became a nightmare and I thought I can't do this. I have to start again. So I am hooked, I'm afraid.*[13]

This is an example of what I call the 'I can't stop and *therefore* I don't want to stop' syndrome. It's actually the other way round.

---

[12] BMJ 2015;350:h1168
[13] http://www.youtube.com/watch?v=B_meK8Dlg5g

What he means, it seems to me, is 'I don't want to stop', and what confirms this belief for him is all the difficulties he finds himself in if he tries, which he attributes to the absence of smoking. So *voilà* – he has an ostensible justification to carry on smoking, which he has continued to do till the present as far as I am aware.

One could also interpret this in a another way: the prospect of stopping smoking is so frightening that he'll make a virtue out of an apparent necessity and aggressively assert his right to harm himself if he chooses.

This he does in a 2013 interview with Stephen Sackur on the BBC Hardtalk programme:

> *So don't tell me that I'm not allowed to smoke in the middle of a fifty acre park in the middle of New York because I'll kill someone, or myself – it's stupid thinking!* [14]

You can see why Mr Irons is such a good actor. When aroused his whole demeanour changes: the angry voice (a bit gravelly but never mind) and the eyes flashing in indignation as he makes his illogical points. Then back to calm and reasonableness when the subject is deftly switched to another on which he has strong views and in which he seems to have had a fair bit of practice: touching women's bottoms. But why is he so edgy and irritable? And he looks awful: the lines and bags only partly hidden by a beard – the typical smoker's face.[15] This is what smoking does to you.

After I had published an earlier article about Jeremy Irons's smoking[16], I felt a bit sorry for him and wrote, care of his publicist, offering my guaranteed successful smoking cessation method. I didn't think it was likely he would take me up on it (he didn't), and I even wondered if he had felt offended at my

---

[14] https://www.youtube.com/watch?v=jg21P6w0Gig
[15] Br Med J (Clin Res Ed) 1985;291:1760
[16] http://tokyobritishclinic.com/articles/?p=115

piece and whether I might hear from his lawyers (I didn't). All that happened was that my letter was ignored.

I do not say any of this to criticise Mr Irons. Rather, I sympathise with him and the countless other smokers who, understandably but mistakenly, think in this way. If you're in this situation the first thing to do is to recognise it and be honest with yourself: 'I don't *really* want to stop.' Then we need to look at this a little more closely.

Obviously it's not because of lack of knowledge of the harm smoking does to you, and I'm not going to remind you of this or the waste of money, etc., because you already know it. Further, although on one level you don't really want to stop, in your heart of hearts you wish you weren't a smoker. So, apart from all the other problems of smoking, every time you light up you're reminded of this conflict.

The key to resolving the conflict, and thereby being able to quit without difficulty, lies in the answer to the question: Why don't you really want to stop smoking?

For the answer, see Appendix.

Chapter 8

Cutting Down Forever

In a medical paper presenting opposing views on the question of whether smokers should be advised to cut down as well as quit[17], almost every sentence on the 'pro' side of the discussion is muddle-headed or just plain wrong.

The opening sentence is: 'Currently, more than half of all smokers in England are trying to reduce the number of cigarettes they smoke.' Then they cite a paper from the US from 2006 which concludes: 'Smoking reduction increases the probability of future cessation.'[18]

This is meaningless. Many smokers when asked about their smoking will say, Yes, they're cutting down, or they're trying to stop. So that's all right then.

Further, the authors regard it as a 'positive behavioural change'. It's not a positive behavioural change; it's a self-delusory excuse to carry on smoking. Some people seem to be cutting down forever. In any case, this is contradicted later in the piece by the statement that 'people are not very successful at cutting down, with reducers smoking only about two cigarettes a day fewer than non-reducers.'

Nonetheless, they think it's useful to encourage more smokers to cut down and to support those who do. Support those who do? How do you do that? Say 'What a good boy/girl you are!' and give them a pat on the head? The Goon Show line, for those old enough to remember it, delivered by a character with the splendidly Dickensian name of Henry Crun, is irresistible: 'Thank you, thank you for your support, I shall always wear it.'

---

[17] BMJ 2014;348:g2787
[18] Nicotine Tob Res 2006;8:739-49.

Smoking is a Psychological Problem

Getting a bit more scientific, they continue:

> *Nicotine addiction leads to neuroadaptation* (changes in the brain) *and cutting down on smoking might reverse some of this, leading to less craving and withdrawal* (what's the difference?)*...Reduction weakens the conditioned response created by smoking, making relapse less likely to be triggered by exposure to cues to smoke after quitting.*

Apart from being pure speculation, this is worse than useless. Smokers don't smoke because of a conditioned response, like Pavlov's dogs, or cues to smoke. They smoke because they become aware of mildly uncomfortable and anxious feelings due to withdrawal of the dose of nicotine provided by the previous cigarette.

Cock-a-doodle-doo! 'It's morning. Time for the first cigarette!' Then, breakfast with coffee. 'I'm having breakfast with coffee, that reminds me, I need another cigarette.' Break at work – another cue – another cigarette! After lunch. 'Ah, I've just finished lunch – time for a fag'. Etc. The smoker is not standing motionless all day in the middle of a room with his eyes closed and his mind a blank. He's always just about to do something, or is in the middle of something or has just finished doing something, whether it's in relation to a meal, taking a break, talking on the phone, drinking a coffee or beer, etc. The cues are purely coincidental. The stimulus for the next cigarette is determined by the time since the last one.

One of my patients told me, 'Stopping smoking is one of the best things I do!' She might have quoted the well-known line of Mark Twain's: 'Giving up smoking is the easiest thing in the world. I know because I've done it thousands of times!'

The afore-mentioned paper concludes: 'Teaching people methods to cut down seems to increase reduction and the chance of achieving cessation.' How patronizing. Do people need to be *taught* how to cut down? It's simple. Smoke one cigarette fewer each day till you've reached zero, for example. Here's another method: smoke one cigarette fewer every two days till you've reached zero. The problem, of course, is what happens when you reach zero, *if* you reach zero? The authors then give up on themselves:

> *Greater promotion of smoking reduction and using nicotine replacement...would mean that more people stop smoking.*

So now we're back to nicotine replacement. What's new? This is:

> *People who are cutting down report that they are doing so mainly with a view to stopping completely.*

Ha ha. And how do they reach that conclusion?

> *We conducted a...telephone survey of 1,000 current daily cigarette smokers...Most smokers (57%) reported previously trying to reduce their smoking, and many (26%) said that they plan to reduce within the next year. Almost half of those planning to quit in the next 12 months (44%) preferred to quit via gradual cessation...*[19]

Ha ha ha. Except it's not funny. How can this be regarded as evidence that cutting down is an aid to quitting? People plan to reduce and quit via gradual cessation, they say. In other words, because of these expressed *intentions* to quit they can feel better about themselves while they carry on smoking for the time being – and how long will that be?

All this sort of advice side-steps or ignores the real or main reason people smoke: *to relieve the temporary discomfort of the*

---

[19] Nicotine and Tobacco Research, 2007, Volume 9, Issue 11, pp1177-1182

withdrawal symptoms of nicotine from the previous cigarette. Once this is understood, it's clear what needs to be done: firstly, stop worrying about all the other supposed reasons for smoking – the cues, associations with a coffee or a meal, stress relief, enjoyment, etc., and, secondly, recognise that the best way of successful quitting is to *stop putting nicotine into your body – by any means.* So, no nicotine maintenance, whether by cutting down, using gum or patches or e-cigarettes, etc.

Chapter 9

Mutiny in the Ranks

A recent article confirms what I've been saying all along: if you're a smoker who wishes to stop you don't need the hindrance of drugs or nicotine maintenance therapy; you don't even need to be talked at for six hours (apart from when you take a cigarette break) in an Allen Carr session (Chapter 12). Some illustrative quotes:

> *Research shows that two-thirds to three-quarters of ex-smokers stop unaided. In contrast, the increasing medicalisation of smoking cessation implies that cessation need be pharmacologically or professionally mediated.*
>
> *In 1986, the American Cancer Society reported that: 'Over 90% of the estimated 37 million people who have stopped smoking in this country since the Surgeon General's first report linking smoking to cancer have done so unaided.'* Today, **unassisted cessation continues to lead the next most successful method (nicotine replacement therapy) by a wide margin.**
>
> ***...paradoxically, the tobacco control community treats this information as if it was somehow irresponsible or subversive.***
>
> *The public is often advised that assistance at least doubles cessation rates...[but] a 1990 US study found 47.5% of those who tried to quit unaided over 10 years were successful, compared with 23.6% using cessation programs...*
>
> *The persistence of unassisted cessation as the most common way that most smokers have succeeded in quitting is an unequivocally positive message...**smokers should be repeatedly told that cold turkey and reducing-then-quitting***

are the methods most commonly used by successful ex-smokers...[20] (Emphasis added.)

The idea that unassisted quitting or cold turkey isn't a bad way to go is taken further in an article entitled *What do we know about unassisted smoking cessation in Australia?*. We are informed of the interesting fact that between 2005 and 2012 in Australia '54% to 69% of ex-smokers quit unassisted and 41% to 58% of current smokers had attempted to quite unassisted.'[21] (Assisted cessation here means using nicotine maintenance therapy or drugs.) The authors seem surprised – even disappointed – that in spite of all the investment in advertising and in making orthodox cessation aids easily available, these are successful in only a minority of smokers who stop or try to stop.

This results from approaching the problem in the wrong way. It's illustrated in a table included in the article which lists, repetitively and rather patronisingly, "Potentially instructive research questions that the Australian research does not currently answer." I'll quote some of these with my comments:

- Why do so many smokers choose not to use assistance in the face of so much persuasion to do so?
  Because they don't really want to stop.
- Why do smokers who quit on their own, perceive assisted cessation to be a sign of weakness?
  Why should they think it's a sign of weakness? Smokers simply get fed up with smoking and just stop, so assistance is irrelevant.

---

[20] The Global Research Neglect of Unassisted Smoking Cessation: Causes and Consequences by Simon Chapman and Ross MacKenzie, PLOS Medicine, February 09, 2010. Doi: 10.1371/journal.pmed.1000216
[21] doi:10.1136/tobaccocontrol-2013-051019

- Do ex-smokers inflate their own role in their quitting and downplay the role assistance played to their success? *Doubtful. Are ex-smokers proud of their success in quitting? If anything they are ashamed they used to smoke.*
- What characterises smokers who want to quit on their own? Is it that they want to quit without pharmacotherapy or without any form of help at all (including help from GPs, quitline services and stop-smoking clinics)?
  This question is pointless. It's the same as asking 'What characterises smokers who want to quit?'
- Have smokers who quit unassisted tried assistance before and realised that motivation and determination are critically important components of quitting?
  The answer is obvious. If you really want to quit, you have really to want to quit, so you do!
- How do those who quit unassisted find the experience in terms of its degree of difficulty?
  This begs the question: it's assumed that if one tries to quit unassisted it will be difficult. Maybe the perceived difficulty is because so many 'experts' who imply that assistance is needed to quit, reinforce the idea that it will be difficult.
- Does the experience of quitting unassisted differ for those who are heavily addicted compared with less addicted smokers?
  This assumes there are degrees of addiction. The idea of being more or less heavily addicted, apart from being wrong, is of no practical relevance and is likely to be counter-productive. If someone is heavily addicted they may think it's too difficult to try to stop. And if someone is less addicted it's not a problem so they needn't try to stop.
- Does the current focus on use of medications to quit mislead smokers about how hard or easy it will be to quit?
  Indeed, it very likely reinforces the perceived difficulty

- of stopping. Smoking- cessation services never suggest it will be easy!
- Have smokers who successfully quit unassisted, previous experience of quitting with assistance? If so, how has this informed their unassisted-quit attempt?
  It sounds as if the authors are desperately trying to find a role for assisted quitting!
- How do those who successfully quit unassisted actually go about doing so?
  Daft question. You stop smoking and thenceforth you're a non-smoker. Or some people may cut down and then stop.
- Is their success linked to deliberate quitting strategies or lifestyle factors (such as exercise, prayer, meditation or diet) that are not used by those who quit with assistance?
  Why make it so complicated? What smokers need to do is to stop. It's not their lifestyles which need changing – it's their smoking!
- Do successful unassisted quitters have common 'meta-narratives' or heuristics that they believe assisted their determination to quit and to not relapse?
  Ditto. And how clever to use such big words! I suppose they mean methods or approaches.
- Is to possible to identify which smokers are likely to quit unassisted, and potentially put in place a spectrum of policy interventions for different types of smokers, which can more effectively and more efficiently help them quit earlier?
  '…potentially put in place a spectrum of policy interventions…' Apart from the awful writing, they can't seem to let go of the idea of the need to 'intervene' in some way.

Unfortunately, the Tobacco Control Industry in the main ignores the results of this kind of research and laments that the numbers attending conventional smoking cessation services are falling. ASH and an organisation calling itself the National Centre for Smoking Cessation and Training, no less, now plead that 'Public Health England must better promote local NHS stop smoking services using mass media campaigns.' [22]

Why does the medical establishment persist in plugging nicotine maintenance and drugs as the best way to stop smoking? It's clear that the best way to stop smoking is – just stop!

---

[22] BMJ 2015;351:h4685.

Chapter 10

Banning Cigarettes

My views on this have been clearly stated in my previous book, but what does the medical literature have to say? Let's look at an editorial in the journal *Tobacco Control* dealing with this matter.[23]

The authors get around to the idea that cigarettes should be banned, sort of:

> ...it is clear that combustible cigarettes should no longer be widely and easily available...the ultimate goal of eradicating use of combustible cigarettes.

They also remind us that:

> ...the commercial manufacture, promotion and sale of cigarettes created an unprecedented industrially produced disease epidemic..[and this] is our biggest and most intractable problem...

Then, with reference to e-cigarettes, they wonder:

> What level of regulation is most appropriate for a product [the e-cigarette] that is likely to be far less deadly than combustible cigarettes, yet is still addictive and may still entail some risk to users is less clear.

Let me try and rewrite this in plain English without all those qualifications of the absolutes:

---

[23] *Tob Control* 2014;23:369-370

Cigarettes are a big problem. It is less clear, however, what level of regulation is appropriate for a product which, though apparently safer than cigarettes, is still addictive and may entail some risk to users.

The article ponderously continues:

> ...it is time to maximise the opportunity [e-cigarettes] may provide to leverage greater regulation of smoked tobacco... Perhaps the greatest contribution these alternative products may ultimately make is in providing further justification for phasing out the most harmful nicotine product: the cigarette.

Why are they so coy about it? Why do we need further justification for phasing out cigarettes? Isn't it enough that they kill 100,000 people in the UK every year?

Another approach is to make it into a kind of game, the 'endgame'.[24] (Comment added.)

> We define a tobacco endgame as initiatives designed to change or permanently eliminate the structural, political, and social dynamics that sustain the tobacco epidemic, so as to achieve, within a specific time, an endpoint for the tobacco epidemic. (Yawn.)

Do they mean, by any chance, the banning of tobacco?

Gaming does, indeed, seem to go on in the dusty recesses of some academic journals. For example, in an editorial, again in *Tobacco Control*, we are informed that 'Endgame thinkers are the visionaries of the tobacco control movement' and can discover 'new endgame ideas for tobacco control'. The writer's approach sounds more like day-dreaming:

---

[24] BMJ 2014;348:g1453

> *Could any of these latest big picture ideas really work? Perhaps not immediately, but they inspire us all to think beyond the next smoke-free ordinance...*[25]

The matter of banning cigarettes is raised, tentatively, in a journal called *Addiction*, as 'Thinking about the unthinkable: a *de facto* prohibition on smoked tobacco products', but this merely discusses phasing out smoked tobacco products as a 'thought experiment'.[26]

Abolishing tobacco is discussed in yet another editorial in *Tobacco Control* under the heading *Questions for a tobacco-free future*.[27] It contains some promising insights:

> *The very phrase 'tobacco control' suggests that tobacco is here to stay...Does tobacco control have any obligation to account for users who 'can't quit'? Do such users even exist?...Tobacco control has learned that aiming too low can be counterproductive...*

Unfortunately, these ideas are not pursued very far and the piece falls flat as it ends on a self-congratulatory note accompanied by crystal ball gazing:

> *Tobacco control advocates have wrought remarkable changes in the last 50 years; the papers in this issue of Tobacco Control suggest that the next 50 years will see even more.*

How many people will die of smoking-related diseases in the next fifty years? We can't wait that long. How about calling for banning cigarettes right now?

---

[25] doi:10.1136/tc.2010.039727
[26] doi:10.1111/j.1360-0443.2007.02129.x
[27] doi:10.1136/tobaccocontrol-2013-051066

At least one other person, Dr Robert N Proctor of Stanford University in the US, argues forcefully for doing this.[28] It's worth quoting his main summary points:

> *The cigarette is the deadliest object in the history of human civilisation. It is also a defective product, a financial burden on cash-strapped societies, an important source of political and scientific corruption, and a cause of both global warming and global warming denial.*
>
> *The most important reason to ban the sale of cigarettes, however, is that most smokers do not even like the fact they smoke; cigarettes are not a recreational drug.*
>
> *It is not in principle difficult to end the sale of cigarettes; most communities–even small towns–could do this virtually overnight. We actually have more power than we realize to put an end this, the world's leading cause of death and disease.*

Is anybody listening?

---

[28] *Why ban the sale of cigarettes? The case for abolition.* doi:10.1136/tobaccocontrol-2012-050811

Chapter 11

World Expert on Smoking and Addiction[29]

With such a billing, who might this be? It's Professor Robert West. He's not a medical doctor but a psychologist, and he thinks unless e-cigarettes are made available we are condemning smokers to death.[30] We shall meet him again in Chapter 15.

I was interested to discover that he published a book in 2013 with the intriguing title *The SmokeFree Formula, A Revolutionary Way to Stop Smoking Now*. Always keen to learn more about helping people to stop smoking, I bought a copy. But there's nothing revolutionary about his approach – it's entirely conventional.

What also struck me about this book is that it's rather pompous and full of unnecessary words, tautologies and repetition, rambling on for 246 pages.

For example, the dedication is not just 'To Susan', but 'To my darling Susan'. Maybe she's a darling to him but why should the reader care?

Then, the acknowledgements, headed 'Thanks Go To…' Why not 'Thanks To…' or simply 'Acknowledgements'? Now he really gets into his hyperbolic stride: 'I am deeply grateful to…' (I am grateful to…); 'Grateful thanks to…' which occurs twice. (Thanks to…) Note he also expresses his grateful thanks to 'several pharmaceutical companies that develop and manufacture smoking cessation treatments for their financial support…' At least we know his competing interests.

---

[29] These words appear on the cover of the book which is reviewed in this chapter.
[30] BBC interview, 28 April 2014. https://www.youtube.com/watch?v=_cqgbdfZk20

Let's move on to the Introduction. There's a subheading: 'Read This First'. Introductions, if they're read at all, are generally read first; that's why they're called introductions.

Unnecessary words: '...by opening this book you have taken a huge stride to giving up smoking forever.' (...you have taken a stride to giving up smoking.); 'I'll then show you how you blend these ingredients together into your own personal formula to be free of smoking forever.' It sounds like a cookery lesson, but presumably he means to say something like: 'I'll then show you how to create a personal formula to be free of smoking.' Still with the cookery theme, illiteracy creeps in: 'What ingredients you choose to use is (*sic*) entirely up to you.' (The ingredients you choose are up to you.)

The worst thing about this introduction, which you are urged to read first, is that it's discouraging to would-be quitters because it emphasises the difficulties they will face:

> *Being bad-tempered is a classic symptom of nicotine withdrawal...There are so many things that could go wrong... incessant cravings...When the going gets tough...*

Professor West bizarrely advises:

> *...you can think of stopping smoking as like* (sic) *looking for love.*

How can you compare looking for love to a wish to stop poisoning yourself with tobacco? He uses this inappropriate analogy to mean you keep trying till you succeed, but why rub it in that it's likely to be so difficult?

At one point he even starts to sound like Jesus:

> *I want this book to be the best investment you ever make. I want you to be healthier, happier and have more money...I*

want to join you in your journey to a better life and be there to help you along the way…I will be with you for as long as it takes…

This passage could be another candidate for inclusion in *Pseuds' Corner* in *Private Eye*.

Reading the first chapter, called 'Understanding Why You Smoke and Find it Hard to Stop', one can begin to understand Professor West's approach. He's done research using questionnaires in which smokers are asked why they smoke and whether they often smoke in certain situations. Also, his team devised the 'Mood and physical symptoms scale questionnaire'. In this his subjects are asked, while smoking and when they've stopped, to rate their feelings over the previous twenty-four hours in terms of depression, anxiety, irritability, restlessness, hunger, poor concentration, poor sleep at night, sores in the mouth, constipation and cough/sore throat. With such leading questions the idea is reinforced that these are symptoms smokers trying to quit may experience.

He does say one sensible thing: 'Your brain has got used to nicotine and is now experiencing withdrawal symptoms because your nicotine level is falling.' Curiously, however, this idea is developed into the theory that

> *…nicotine has trained that part of your brain that gets you to do things to light up a cigarette whenever you find yourself in a situation where you would normally smoke.*

Not quite clear about that. However, the reason this happens, he says, is that nicotine causes dopamine to be released in your brain 'which acts as a kind of reward' and:

> *It is this dopamine release that attaches the impulse to smoke to whatever situation you happen to be in when you normally do it.*

Geddit?

So much for the science. The writing is patronising:

> ...these nerve cells need to talk to each other...Nicotine is like a cuckoo in the nest...your brain is being taught to sit up and beg for nicotine...smoking a cigarette is a bit like eating food when you are hungry, drinking when you are thirsty, telling a funny joke (Would you tell an unfunny joke?)...This chemical is called acetylcholine. (Don't worry, I'm not going to test you on these names later!)

The discouragement continues:

> ...nicotine...has changed your brain chemistry to create powerful **urges** to smoke...you will have to show self-control... exert self-control and fight off the urge to smoke...you still need willpower...you start to feel a whole load of unpleasant symptoms when you can't smoke...nicotine withdrawal symptoms come on very quickly and they are not pleasant. (Emphasis in original.)

And so on, and on.

The next two chapters are dumbed-down lessons in the psychology of smoking and addiction, respectively. Among other gems the author self-effacingly mentions:

> ...since you are so engrossed in my lesson in psychology... When I was first at university it took me a year to discover I didn't really like staying up all night and partying...

Well, fancy that! A hint of doubt on this confession does seem to creep in since he asks the reader, and presumably himself, 'What am I saying here?' Indeed.

Chapter 4, 'Why Do You Want to Stop Smoking?', does equally well in the boredom stakes, opening with 'I've talked a lot about how nicotine keeps you smoking.' Yes, he has. And more illiteracy: 'Do you have a smokers' (*sic*) cough?'

Let's move on to Part Two, subtitled with our now familiar cookery theme, 'The Ingredients'. The reader is invited to 'Think of this section as a storehouse full of useful ingredients sitting on shelves waiting for you to use them.' (The last word is redundant.) Then he goes into the different types of evidence of effectiveness in helping people to stop smoking including the hallowed Randomised Controlled Trial.

The trouble with this book, in my view, is that it's based on the false premise that smoking cessation is suitable to be investigated by the same methods used in the scientific study of the treatment of disease. For example, it you suffer from a stomach ulcer, this can be treated with drug A or drug B and a randomised controlled trial can be done to see which, if either, is better. But smoking is an entirely voluntary activity. All the smoker has to do, if he or she wants to, is to *stop smoking*.

Unfortunately, and in my experience wrongly, many statements in this book indicate that it's very *very* hard to stop smoking without using nicotine products and/or drugs. Presumably Professor West makes this assertion on the grounds of his research and on randomised controlled trials of different smoking cessation methods. However, in spite of the scientific veneer, I contend these results are likely to be of little benefit for real people who smoke.

He also describes his 'Nicotine withdrawal: The train study', which he conducted with Professor Peter Hajek, modestly introduced as the 'founder of the model of group support given to smokers right across the globe', whose other claim to fame is his assertion that vaping is no more harmful than drinking coffee.[31] No citation is given, but apparently they took a group of thirty smokers and put them on a non-smoking train from London to Glasgow.

---

[31] BBC interview, 28 April 2014. https://www.youtube.com/watch?v=_cqgbdfZk20

> *We then measured how they felt every 30 minutes during the four-hour journey. This was the first study anyone had ever done to see how quickly nicotine withdrawal symptoms and urges to smoke emerged in a natural setting…*

(The words 'anyone had ever done' are redundant.) It's hardly a natural setting. Thirty smokers making an otherwise pointless train journey used a tick-box method to try to answer the above-mentioned question. Not surprisingly

> *We found that the mood of our volunteers started to deteriorate quite quickly, and…continued to get progressively worse…When the train reached Glasgow our volunteers couldn't wait to get off the train and light up.*

And the conclusion of this trial?

> *Nicotine withdrawal symptoms come on very quickly and they are not pleasant.*

What a waste of thirty London-to-Glasgow return train fares. This depressing result was entirely predictable. But I suppose the mention of this and similar experiments is only to be expected in a book written by a professor of psychology who does research rather than who actually treats smokers. (I asked Professor West if he had treated any smokers himself; he said he had, but declined to say how many or to enter into a discussion.)

This kind of research is very different from the approach where individual smokers are asked open-ended questions about what they feel when they haven't smoked for a while or have tried to stop. In my experience it's striking that most people find it difficult to say anything at all, other than that they feel they want a cigarette.

Smoking is a Psychological Problem

Let's continue with our review of the book. Chapter 7, subtitled 'Your Approach', we are patronisingly told '...is all about you.' This nice warm feeling, however, is quickly dispelled by yet another exposition of all the problems you are likely to encounter when you stop smoking:

> ***The first four weeks*** *are definitely the hardest from the point of view of cravings and withdrawal symptoms. There may well be times when you are hanging on by the skin of your teeth. You will need to do everything you can to keep from having that fateful puff on a cigarette...**The next four weeks** are easier... but if you are still finding it hard and your morale is sagging, things can be very difficult...**After that**...You may well miss your cigarettes...It's just sooo* (sic) *easy to pick up a cigarette and smoke it.* (Emphasis in original.)

Gee, thanks Professor.

I'll quote just one more specimen of dumbing down: '...the bit of your brain that is giving you the urges to smoke is not the clever part. It's the stupid part.'

He is also at pains to stress that if you don't stop smoking 'you have not failed – there is no such thing as failure when it comes to trying to stop smoking.' Well, that's a funny way of looking at it. The definition of a smoker could be someone who has failed to stop: this is demonstrated every time he or she lights another cigarette.

Chapter 12

What About Allen Carr?

If you look into how to stop smoking you may come upon the name of Allen Carr. In fact, his name used to come up in discussions with some of my patients who wanted to quit. They had read his book and a few had attended his group sessions, but they were still smoking.

Allen Carr died in 2006, ironically from lung cancer, but his organization continues and claims over 90% success from their 'Easyway' method. This is on the basis that only 10% of clients ask for their money back, but it's a poor indicator of success. People who have failed to quit may feel too embarrassed to ask for their money back.

I obtained a copy of the 4th edition of his *Easy Way to Stop Smoking*.[32] It's written from the perspective of the author's experience as a claimed former one-hundred-a-day smoker. The book is over-long (206 pages) and repetitive. Much of it is taken up with an exposition of why one shouldn't smoke, as if he's trying to *persuade* smokers they should stop. The writing is sexist, smokers nearly always being referred to with masculine pronouns. There are numerous stylistic and grammatical infelicities, e.g., '...this explanation explains why...' and 'It started with just Joyce and I at home...'

Many of the medical aspects of the effects of smoking are crudely, inaccurately and repetitively stated:

> *The 'gunge' never leaves your body completely. (p34)*
> *...the progressive gunging up of our arteries and veins and the gradual starving of every muscle and organ of our*

---
[32] Penguin Books, 2009.

bodies of oxygen and nutrients and replacing them with poisons and carbon monoxide... (p79)

...the gradual and progressive deterioration of our immune system caused by this gunging-up process...How can your immune system work effectively when you are starving every muscle and organ of oxygen and nutrients and replacing them with carbon monoxide and poisons? (p80)

...this progressive process of gunging-up and starvation of oxygen and nutrients... (p86)

The progressive blocking up of the arteries and veins with poison starves the brain of oxygen. (p53)

...the cigarette not only destroys your nerves but is a powerful poison... (p49)

...smoking gradually destroys your immune system. (p81)

...smoking coagulates the blood...and the brownish red colour was due to lack of oxygen. (p82)

Although he has intuitively grasped why people smoke – because of nicotine addiction and withdrawal symptoms – this is merely repeated frequently and he falls into simplistic layman's expressions:

The little monster inside your stomach...the big monster in the mind. (pp98-99)

Think of the little monster as a sort of tapeworm inside your stomach. (p158)

What you are trying to achieve when you quit smoking is to kill both the little nicotine monster in your body and the big monster inside your brain... (p168)

He can't refrain from using crude scare tactics:

...a whole filthy lifetime of spending a small fortune just for the privilege of destroying yourself physically and mentally, a lifetime of slavery, a lifetime of bad breath. (p110)

Cigarettes...are filth and poison...the drug begins to destroy you physically and mentally. (p119)
...it helps to force as many of the filthy things down your throat as possible. (p130)
...filthy drug addiction. (p196)
...destroying himself physically and mentally...facing a lifetime of filth, bad breath and stained teeth. (p138)
Inhale the filth deeply into your lungs...put these filthy things in my mouth... (p180)
[Smoking] is drug addiction, a disease and Number 1 killer in society. (p130)
[The cigarette] happens to be the Number 1 killer poison in society. (p156)
Smoking is by far the biggest killer in society... (p202)

With regard to his group sessions, I've learnt these go on for six hours with regular smoking breaks. Presumably the group leaders don't want the clients to be distracted from being talked at for so long by their cravings for a cigarette. I disagree with this approach. Apart from the undesirability of smoking even *one* extra cigarette, I invite patients to use the feelings of nicotine withdrawal they experience during the session, if any, to help them *demonstrate to themselves* the mechanism of addiction.

Being able to articulate these feelings – not just having them told to you by someone else – is central to successful and easy smoking cessation.

What this book lacks, probably because Mr Carr didn't have the necessary medical or biological knowledge, is a clear explanation about the mechanism of addiction, how this makes smokers want to keep on smoking and how to use this knowledge to stop without difficulty.

PART TWO

Harm Reduction

Chapter 13

Smoking Harm Reduction – a Flawed Concept

As I pointed out in my earlier book, it's not as if smoking is a natural disaster, like floods or tuberculosis, for which there's no realistic prospect of eradication in the foreseeable future, and therefore the best that can be done is to try to mitigate these serious problems. Smoking, on the other hand, is an *un*natural disaster – entirely man-made and unnecessary. In theory, all that needs to be done is to ban the sale of tobacco products and the vast majority of smokers would, perforce, stop. Alas, at present the political will to do this is lacking.

So what's wrong with the so-called harm-reduction approach in the meantime?

What's wrong with it is that it doesn't take properly into account the fact that smoking is legalised drug addiction – the drug, of course, being nicotine. It's true that harm reduction is the aim in some other areas of medical practice, in particular, heroin addiction. For registered addicts a prescription drug called methadone can be taken by mouth and appears less harmful than continuing to inject heroin – which is a killer. But it's used under medical supervision and by only a small number of heroin addicts.

In the Tobacco Control Industry, however, harm reduction is the nihilistic concept that it is, or should be, public policy that millions of people would be walking around addicted to the poison nicotine in a supposedly less harmful way than smoking. This might be a half-way stage if tobacco were banned (or a ban gradually phased in) *at the same time*, but nobody apart from me and one or two other courageous individuals seems to want to advocate such a step!

What's also wrong with harm reduction is that it perpetuates the idea that nicotine addiction is terribly hard to get out of. Therefore, if smokers can't or won't stop smoking, they should be encouraged to use nicotine patches/gum/tablets/inhalers or e-cigarettes instead of, or in addition to, cigarettes.

Such an approach fails to take on board the fact that smokers are all (or nearly all) in the same boat: they apparently can't or don't want to quit. Or it may be rationalisation: the previously mentioned 'I can't quit and *therefore* I don't want to quit' syndrome. This is the central problem with smoking. Of course, if you do surveys you might get a result showing something like 'two thirds of smokers say they want to quit'. But as I also pointed out in my earlier book, depending on how you put the question, the result can show that 100% of smokers want to quit or that 100% of smokers don't want to quit.

Even among smokers who say they want to quit, the reality is that most of them don't *really* want to quit; that's why they're smokers. And this is the reason why, in spite of the wide availability and promotion of apparently less harmful nicotine delivery devices, there are still about ten million adult smokers in Britain[33], about 42.1 million smokers in the US[34] and more than one billion smokers worldwide[35].

Another objection to smoking harm reduction is that it implies smoking can be regarded as a disease – which manifestly it is not.

Let's consider some real diseases. For example, there's a disorder called atrial fibrillation in which the heart beats irregularly. This can result in blood clots forming in the heart and being carried to the brain to cause strokes. Sometimes the abnormal rhythm can be cured, but if it can't, it's perfectly

---

[33] http://ash.org.uk/files/documents/ASH_106.pdf   Accessed 24 August 2015.
[34] http://www.cdc.gov/tobacco/data_statistics/fact_sheets/adult_data/cig_smoking/ Accessed 24 August 2015.
[35] WHO fact sheet No. 339, July 2015.

reasonable to talk of harm reduction by prescribing anticoagulants (drugs to make the blood less likely to clot). Though not completely safe, it's been shown in many scientific trials that such patients are significantly less likely to suffer harm by using these drugs than if they don't.

Another example is type II diabetes, which tends to affect overweight adults who may have no symptoms, at least during the early stages of the disease. If nothing is done they may suffer serious problems affecting the eyes, kidneys and blood vessels. The use of drugs is generally justified in these patients, the aim being to reduce the risk of harm which is otherwise likely.

It needs to be stressed that smoking is not a naturally occurring illness like atrial fibrillation or diabetes, and even though the result is often fatal, it's strange to consider it as a disease in the usual sense of the word. After all, it's entirely in the hands of the smoker whether to smoke or not. The cure is simple: stop smoking – and don't start again. This being the case, why is it that the attitude of many doctors towards smoking seems to be that it will never be possible to get everyone to stop, so the best we can do is encourage smokers to smoke fewer cigarettes or use a less harmful nicotine delivery device, or both.

Why aim so low? Instead of putting so much effort into harm reduction, what about striving to achieve harm *abolition* by banning the sale of cigarettes and nicotine products?

Chapter 14

Harm Reduction and the Emperor's New Clothes

For another view of the problem, let's look at a paper issued by NICE in June 2013 entitled *Tobacco: harm reduction approaches to smoking*. At first glance this looks like it could be a good idea, but then we're confronted with this:

> *This guidance is about helping people, particularly those who are highly dependent on nicotine, who:*
> - *may not be able (or do not want) to stop smoking in one step*
> - *may want to stop smoking, without necessarily giving up nicotine*
> - *may not be ready to stop smoking, but want to reduce the amount they smoke.*[36]

All smokers are dependent on the poison nicotine. This could serve as a definition of a smoker. The qualification 'highly' is superfluous: if someone's addicted, they're addicted. As indicated in Chapter 9 and explained in detail in my earlier book, the concept of degrees of addiction is pointless and counterproductive. Further, it's of no help and patronizing for smokers to be regarded as so feeble they 'may not be able or do not want or may not be ready to stop smoking', or as 'wanting to stop smoking without necessarily giving up nicotine'.

The problem is that most smokers don't understand that they smoke only for the relief of nicotine withdrawal symptoms. Typically, they think they smoke because of habit, stress relief, enjoyment

---
[36] guidance.nice.org.uk/ph45

(especially after a meal, with an alcoholic drink or a coffee, first thing in the morning, etc.) or as an aid to concentration, among other specious reasons. Further, the smoking public is not helped by doctors who put about the idea that although the main reason for smoking is nicotine addiction, people *also* smoke because of the release of dopamine and stimulation of the pleasure centre in the brain, because the brain is altered in smokers, because smokers seek the stimulant and relaxing effects (ignoring the contradiction) of nicotine or because of the 'cues' to smoke, etc.

It seems that the harm-reducers, being unable to understand that smoking *is* nicotine addiction, are not in a position to undeceive smokers about their illusions. Therefore, the thinking goes, nicotine is needed in some form or other to perpetuate the illusion of it being enjoyable or helpful. So we need safer delivery devices for the poison nicotine!

Let's look at this paper in a little more detail. (My comments in parentheses):

> *…smoking is highly addictive largely because it delivers nicotine very quickly to the brain and this makes stopping smoking difficult* (Then why are some people addicted to nicotine gum or patches or vaping? The speed of delivery of nicotine to the brain, of itself, isn't why people are addicted.)

> *…nicotine levels in licensed nicotine-containing products are much lower than in tobacco, and the way these products deliver nicotine makes them less addictive than smoking tobacco.* (Addiction is addiction; it's unhelpful to talk of degrees of addiction.)

> *…there is reason to believe that lifetime use of licensed nicotine-containing products will be considerably less harmful than smoking.* (Why would anyone in their right mind want to use any form of nicotine at all, ever, let alone for a lifetime?)

Smoking is a Psychological Problem

If someone does not want, is not ready or is unable to stop smoking in one step, ask if they would like to consider a harm-reduction approach. If they agree, help them to identify why they smoke, their smoking triggers and their smoking behaviour. (It would be hard to think of a more feeble approach to smoking cessation. In any case, it's of no help to consider smoking triggers and behaviour as if these are something separate from the addiction.)

Advise people that they can continue to use licensed nicotine-containing products in the long term, rather than risk relapsing after they have stopped, or reduced their smoking. (Is it a kindness to indulge smokers in this way? Any use of nicotine is pointless and potentially harmful.)

If more intensive support is required, offer a referral to stop smoking services. These services provide pharmacotherapies and more comprehensive support. (This means nicotine maintenance or prescription drugs to suppress withdrawal symptoms – unnecessary and counterproductive.)

Find out about the person's smoking behaviour and level of nicotine dependence by asking how many cigarettes they smoke – and how soon after waking. (Again, the unhelpful and illogical concept of the level of nicotine dependence.)

Help people who are aiming to reduce the amount they smoke (but not intending to stop) to set a date when they will have achieved their goal. Help them to develop a schedule for this or to identify specific periods of time (or specific events) when they will not smoke. (It does little or nothing for your health if you continue to smoke reduced amounts.)

> *Tell people who are not prepared to stop smoking that the health benefits from smoking reduction are unclear. However, advise them that if they reduce their smoking now they are more likely to stop smoking in the future. Explain that this is particularly true if they use licensed nicotine-containing products to help reduce the amount they smoke.* (What a cop-out! It's saying reduced smoking is all right because you'll be likely to stop in the future. Many smokers say they plan to stop in the future. As a smoker, your need is to stop right now.)

> *People often try many times before they eventually succeed in stopping smoking. People who have recently tried and failed are more likely to try again – but they are also more likely to relapse than those who have not tried recently. Relapse is associated with:*
> - *nicotine dependence*
> - *exposure to smoking cues*
> - *craving*
> - *withdrawal symptoms*
> - *lack of help to stop (the latter could include medication, behavioural support or support from family and friends)*

Let me try and rewrite the last paragraph in plain English and get rid of the bulleted list:

> 'People who smoke may be considered as having failed to stop. If smokers stop for a while but relapse, this is because when they stop they may believe any withdrawal symptoms they experience are insupportable. It's convenient to blame this on lack of help in stopping. It's like saying someone falls over because no-one caught her by the arm.'

The expression 'harm reduction' is seductive. It enables those in the Tobacco Control Industry to feel good about themselves in spite of having nothing better to offer. 'Look', they seem be saying, 'smoking is harmful and can cause lung cancer and heart disease, but if you use these *licensed* nicotine-containing products then you'll do yourself less harm than if you continue to smoke.' So why has there not been wholesale uptake of these licensed reduced-harm ways of poisoning yourself with nicotine? Part of the reason could be that smokers don't want to admit to themselves every time they light up that they are doing themselves harm. They don't think of cigarettes in that way most of the time. After all, cigarettes can be picked up as part of the weekly grocery shopping! Smokers, when they feel the urge to smoke, without necessarily being aware of it, just look forward to feeling better – having the 'urge' quickly relieved after lighting up. Their subjective experience is at variance with the horrible picture and warning on the packet: 'Yes, I know it's bad for me, but I do so enjoy a cigarette!'

Furthermore, these *licensed* nicotine-containing products are presented in a negative way: harm reduction. Can you imagine any other consumer product being promoted like this?

> 'Eat Muckdonald's hamburgers with reduced fat! They're less likely to raise your cholesterol and cause a heart attack than eating Greaseburger King's hamburgers!'

As I pointed out in the previous chapter, promotion of alternative nicotine delivery devices might make sense *if cigarettes were banned at the same time*, and it would help smokers to recognize that they smoke only because of drug addiction. But the promoters of *licensed* nicotine-containing products skirt around this essential message and instead imply something like this:

'If you fail to stop smoking you haven't really failed because the reason you still smoke is due to nicotine dependence *and* exposure to smoking cues *and* cravings *and* withdrawal symptoms *and* lack of help with which to stop, including medication, behavioural support or support from family and friends.'

The Emperor has no clothes, or at any rate very few clothes. Why are those in the Tobacco Control Industry so lacking in confidence or blinded by their own science that they can't put out a simple message such as the following?

- You smoke *only* because you are addicted to the poison nicotine
- This shows itself by *withdrawal symptoms* shortly after you take a dose of nicotine by smoking a cigarette
- Withdrawal symptoms consist of mild anxiety or nervousness
- It is the relief of these symptoms by the next cigarette, that is, by the next dose of the poison nicotine, which creates the *illusion* of pleasure or relaxation
- If you do not take any more nicotine into your body, what will happen to the withdrawal symptoms?
- They will go away!
- And never come back – unless you put more of the poison nicotine into your body
- And another thing…
- Er…That's it![37]

---

[37] With apologies to *Private Eye*.

Chapter 15

Condemning People to Death

The World Health Organisation (WHO) recommends that governments should regulate electronic cigarettes (e-cigarettes) and support research into their safety and efficacy in smoking cessation.[38] Following this lead the British government has decided to regulate them as medicines from May 2016.

This is curious. Why should e-cigarettes be regulated as medicines? They're not medicines and I can't see the logic of treating them as such as long as vendors make no health claims.

Nicotine has no recognised medicinal use – unless one stretches the concept to include the idea that it may help you to stop smoking if you take it into your body in a different way. All that e-cigarettes do is enable the user to absorb relatively pure nicotine without the thousands of other chemicals you cannot avoid also inhaling by smoking cigarettes.

Incidentally, what does it mean, efficacy? In the medical sense it means the ability of a drug to produce a desired effect. What is this desired effect? Is it an orgasmic sensation or a vision of heaven? I think not. It probably means that it satisfies the user's need for another dose of the poison nicotine, which is to say it *relieves the temporary discomfort of the withdrawal symptoms of the previous dose* – a self-perpetuating situation. And what's the good of that? A short time later the symptoms come back, so you want another dose, and the cycle repeats indefinitely.

One enthusiast for e-cigarettes whom we met earlier, the self-styled world expert on smoking and addiction, Professor Robert West, gets a bit carried away, saying:

---

[38] http://www.who.int/nmh/events/2014/backgrounder-e-cigarettes/en/

Condemning People to Death

> *You kind of have to be crazy to carry on smoking a conventional cigarette when e-cigarettes are available...If we fail to take this opportunity that electronic cigarettes are potentially providing then we're really condemning people to death.*[39]

Condemning people to death? Do we line them up against a wall or string them up from lamp-posts? What I guess he means is that if we (whoever 'we' are: the medical profession, the health service, the so-called tobacco control community or the government?) fail to take this opportunity, etc., then you, the smoker, are going to die because e-cigarettes are not available because of unprogressive legislation or because the health community thought they were dangerous when they weren't.

Perhaps we should take into account Professor West's competing interests. In addition to those mentioned in Chapter 11, he has a share of a patent for a novel nicotine delivery device and is a trustee of an organisation called QUIT. This organisation promotes nicotine products and stop smoking drugs; it wrongly and discouragingly states that only 3% of smokers succeed by willpower alone.[40]

What an extraordinary idea. Because we don't all rush to embrace e-cigarettes, many unfortunate smokers who are suffering from the incurable disease of smoking will die. But all they have to do, to avoid an untimely death from this cause, is to STOP SMOKING (unless they've left it too late). Unfortunately, Professor West seems to takes the nihilistic view that the only thing we can do to save lives is to enable smokers to absorb the poison nicotine into their bodies in an apparently less harmful way.

Writing in favour of regulating e-cigarettes is Simon Chapman, Professor of Public Health at the University of Sydney.

---

[39] BBC interview, 28 April 2014. https://www.youtube.com/watch?v=_cqgbdfZk20
[40] http://www.quit.org.uk/stop-smoking-products

He has an impressive list of publications to his name but as far as I can see doesn't have a medical qualification and I doubt he's treated a single patient for nicotine addiction. 'Tobacco use may kill a billion people this century' he warns, and he thinks this is due to 'governments failing to regulate this dangerous consumer product'.[41]

Here we have the problem in a nutshell. Cigarettes are not a normal consumer product. They should be seen for what they are: legalized addictive drug delivery devices.

Professor Chapman, however, believes there is a need 'to study large populations and build the evidence about whether e-cigarettes do accelerate quitting.' This is in spite of citing a preliminary study which showed there were no differences in quit rates between e-cigarette users and non-users.[42] So, more studies. That should keep him busy for a while and clock up yet more learned papers. Further, he advocates that nicotine users should have to have some form of licence in the same way that patients require a prescription for drugs in the treatment of illness.

What he doesn't seem to understand is that *nicotine products don't need to be regulated; they need to be got rid of.*

He goes on to say that 'e-cigarettes may in fact turn out to be a Trojan horse, stimulating regulators to take more seriously the regulation of all tobacco nicotine products'. This repetitive sentence shows confusion about ancient history. The Greek gift of the wooden horse *failed* to stimulate the defenders of Troy to take more seriously suspicions that the horse might not have been what it seemed; the doubters were over-ruled and the city was destroyed. Or does Professor Chapman mean that e-cigarettes, or at any rate un-regulated e-cigarettes, may undermine and even reverse tobacco control gains so far achieved? If, on the other hand, he means that the advent of e-cigarettes could be

---

[41] BMJ 2013;346:f3840
[42] Am J Prev Med 2013;44:207-15

an opportunity to regulate ordinary cigarettes out of existence, I would be all for it. But he doesn't. I once asked him to explain to me why cigarettes should not be banned; all he offered in reply was a cliché: 'Because politics is the art of the possible.'[43]

If e-cigarettes are regulated, what will this mean in practice? They will be available to people – over a certain age, presumably, and maybe on a prescription or licence and perhaps with some other restrictions – who wish to use them as a new nicotine delivery device. And what good will that do?

It still doesn't seem to be generally understood that if you put the poison nicotine into your body by whatever means – conventional cigarettes, e-cigarettes, or nicotine gum, patches or suppositories – you will likely want to keep doing it.

Even so, it would be nice to think that the poison nicotine of itself, at least in the small dose provided by a puff of an e-cigarette, would be harmless. But what if you do this repeatedly every day, for years or even decades? Professor Chapman raises the concern that it may not be so benign to baste one's lungs with nicotine and fine particles 150 times a day, or about 55,000 times a year, these being the typical numbers of puffs which a 'vaper' is likely to take.[44]

It's a good point because, after all, the function of the lungs is gaseous exchange – absorbing oxygen and exhaling carbon dioxide – not to absorb noxious chemicals into the bloodstream and deposit fine particles into the alveoli (the deepest recesses of the lungs).

The above-mentioned WHO report also says:

> ...*existing evidence shows that e-cigarette aerosol is not merely "water vapour" as is often claimed in the marketing of these products. While they are likely to be less toxic than*

---

[43] Simon Chapman: personal communication.
[44] BMJ 2014;349:g5512

conventional cigarettes, e-cigarette use poses threats to adolescents and foetuses of pregnant mothers using these devices...E-cigarettes also increase the exposure of non-smokers and bystanders to nicotine and a number of toxicants...

That should give one pause for thought.

In any case, the idea that e-cigarettes can be helpful in smoking cessation is controversial. Why should they be any more successful than nicotine gum or patches? The hope seems to be that current smokers will stop smoking or smoke fewer cigarettes, but there's a risk they may continue long-term to use e-cigarettes – with their as yet unknown risks – instead of, or in addition to, conventional cigarettes. Furthermore, obviously, curious and impressionable young people may well be tempted to try e-cigarettes and this may lead to them smoking when they otherwise wouldn't have done.

This is indeed a problem according to a study done at the University of California:

> Use of e-cigarettes does not discourage, and may encourage, conventional cigarette use among US adolescents...e-cigarette use is aggravating rather than ameliorating the tobacco epidemic among youth...some are introduced to the addictive drug nicotine through e-cigarettes...[45]

Well, blow me down.

---

[45] http://archpedi.jamanetwork.com/article.aspx?articleid=1840772

Chapter 16

E-Cigarette Circus

Following on from their muddle-headed report in 2007, *Harm reduction in nicotine addiction; helping people who can't quit*, the Royal College of Physicians (RCP) of the UK in June 2014 issued a new statement on e-cigarettes.[46]

After the usual mantra drawing attention once again to the tragic fact that 'Tobacco is still the UK's biggest public health issue, causing 100,000 deaths per year', and throwing in the distressing further information that 'For every death caused by smoking, approximately twenty smokers are suffering from a smoking-related disease', the RCP now feels that 'The emergence and rapid growth in the use of electronic cigarettes since the [2007] report was published require a specific policy statement on their use'.

So here they go (paraphrasing slightly):

- *The RCP recognises that electronic cigarettes can provide an effective, affordable and readily available alternative to conventional cigarettes.*
- *The RCP advocates proportionate regulation to maximise the overall public health benefit.*
- *Regulation should ensure that products deliver nicotine effectively and safely; that advertising and promotion do not target young people or other non-smokers; and that advertising and use (for example, in public places) do not undermine smoking prevention policies.*
- *The RCP believes that e-cigarettes could lead to significant falls in the prevalence of smoking in the UK, prevent many*

---

[46] See Chapter 14 of my *Stop Smoking: Real Help at Last*. YouCaxton Publications, 2014.

deaths and help to reduce the social inequalities in health that tobacco smoking currently exacerbates.

These aspirations seem based on wish-fulfilment rather than proven facts, and I find it hard to believe the anonymous author wasn't laughing up his sleeve when he wrote this. What do they mean 'deliver nicotine effectively and safely'? Reminiscent of the days when milk was delivered daily in bottles to your doorstep, they're referring to nicotine delivery devices, neglecting to explain why nicotine should be available at all, anyway, anyhow. Aren't there enough problems already with illicit drugs?

Jumping on the bandwagon, Public Health England (part of the Department of Health of the UK) in 2015 issued a report called *E-cigarettes: an evidence update*.[47] The lead author is one Ann McNeill who, in these days of super-specialization, is a Professor of Tobacco Addiction in the National Addiction Centre. We'll come back to her in a moment.

Another author is our old friend Professor Peter 'nicotine-itself-is-harmless' Hajek[48] who, though he denies links with any e-cigarette manufacturer, has received research funding from and provided consultancy to manufacturers of stop-smoking medications.

The report urges that e-cigarettes be promoted by stop-smoking services as one of the 'tools' for smoking cessation. It also declares that e-cigarettes are 'at least 95% less harmful than tobacco.' I wonder how they worked that out, and what does it mean anyway? Importantly, they also 'found no evidence that e-cigarettes acted as a route into smoking for children and non-smokers.'

Unfortunately, this last assertion is contradicted by a paper in the *Journal of the American Medical Association* which concluded:

---
[47] www.gov.uk/government/publications/e-cigarettes-an-evidence-update
[48] https://www.youtube.com/watch?v=SVS0_BGHHjM

> *Among high school students in Los Angeles, those who had ever used e-cigarettes...compared with nonusers were more likely to report initiation of combustible tobacco use over the next year.*[49]

This is one of the main problems with e-cigarettes.

Apart from that, the Public Health England report was strongly criticized in an editorial in the prestigious medical journal *The Lancet,* which pointed out that the report's conclusions were based on a study of 'the opinions of a small group of individuals with no prespecified expertise in tobacco control'.[50]

It turns out that this study was led by the well-named and eccentric Dr David Nutt, who was dismissed in 2009 as chair of the government's Advisory Council on the Misuse of Drugs after saying that ecstasy, cannabis and LSD are less dangerous than alcohol and tobacco. Furthermore, two of the portly Dr Nutt's colleagues are mentioned in *The Lancet* editorial as having potential conflicts of interest due to their associations with an e-cigarette distributor and manufacturers of smoking cessation products, respectively.

The British Medical Journal also waded in with an aptly titled article, *Evidence about electronic cigarettes: a foundation built on rock or sand?*[51] Firstly, the authors remind us that:

> *Where there is uncertainty about risks, the precautionary principle should apply. Thus, in the absence of scientific consensus that the substance is not harmful to the public, the burden of proof that it is not harmful falls on those taking an action.*

---

[49] JAMA. 2015;314(7):700-707
[50] http://www.thelancet.com/journals/lancet/article/PIIS0140-6736%2815%2900042-2/fulltext
[51] BMJ 2015;351:h4863

Then they point out a number of potential serious problems with these devices (paraphrased):

- There is concern about the uptake of e-cigarettes among people, especially children and adolescents, who would not otherwise smoke.
- The long term health effects of e-cigarettes are unknown.
- E-cigarettes contain substances such as formaldehyde which can cause cancer, as well as various flavourings and other substances which may be harmful to health.
- If e-cigarettes are used to reduce smoking, as opposed to quitting, there may be no overall benefit for health.
- One study shows that dual use (smoking and vaping) was above 80% after 12 months follow-up.
- There is no evidence which clearly shows that e-cigarettes are as effective as established quitting aids for smoking.
- Evidence on the risk of e-cigarette aerosol to bystanders (second-hand vaping) in enclosed public spaces is sparse, and it may be premature to claim there is no risk.

The article also mentions a systematic review (a study of other studies) of December 2014 which makes very interesting reading and is worth quoting in some detail.[52] The two Danish authors looked at seventy-six studies which investigated e-cigarettes. Their bottom line was that:

- No firm conclusions can be drawn on the safety of electronic cigarettes.
- The findings in the seventy-six studies were often inconsistent and contradicting.

---

[52] Pisinger C, Døssing M. *A systematic review of health effects of electronic cigarettes* doi:10.1016/j.ypmed.2014.10.009

- Serious methodological problems were identified and there is no long-term follow-up.
- In 34% of the articles the authors had a conflict of interest.
- Electronic cigarettes can hardly be considered harmless.

Furthermore, it's of great concern that many of these studies found contaminants and other potentially harmful substances in the vapour produced by e-cigarettes:

> *One puff of e-cigarette vapor contained numerous particles, mainly tin, silver, nickel and aluminum...Tin, chromium, and nickel were found as nano-particles...Another study found cadmium, nickel and lead in almost all vapors of twelve brands but the amounts of toxic metals were low...Some studies found tobacco-specific nitrosamines (which can cause cancer)...In one study the potential human carcinogens formaldehyde, acetaldehyde and acrolein were detected in the vapors of almost all e-cigarettes...Volatile organic compounds such as toluene and p,m-xylene were identified in almost all vapors... carcinogenic polycyclic aromatic hydrocarbons in indoor air increased by 20% after vaping...One study found potentially harmful additives, such as coumarin...Products advertised as containing tadalafil contained amino-tadalafil (used to treat erectile dysfunction). Products advertised as containing rimonabant (an appetite suppressant drug withdrawn from the market due to potentially serious side effects), contained rimonabant plus an oxidative impurity of rimonabant. One study found significant amounts of silicate beads in the aerosol.* (Paraphrased and references removed for readability.)

Of course, Professor Ann McNeill was not going to take this lying down. She became very cross at all this criticism of her 'e-cigarettes are at least 95% less harmful than tobacco' claim, especially at *The British Medical Journal* article which she called 'offensive'[53]. This is rather strong language for professional intercourse; one might disagree or suggest a colleague is mistaken, but it's another matter to take criticism personally.

I ask the reader's indulgence while I make a slight digression to get a feel for Professor McNeill's activities at the National Addiction Centre. This institution modestly describes itself as '… one of the most productive addictions research groups in Europe. We represent one of the chosen areas of important health-related study…' In the list of publications mentioned on its website for 2014 Professor McNeill was a co-author of twenty-two papers, which means one churned out in just over every two weeks. In none of these was she the sole author, the number of contributors varying between two and nineteen. Therefore, on average she collaborated with nearly seven other people for each paper. What, I wonder, were her exact contributions to them all? It reminded me of the joke about animal experiments: the rat is an animal which, when injected, produces a paper.

Now the plot thickens. Would you believe it, there is a recently formed organization (surprisingly, a registered charity) in the UK whose name says it all: *The New Nicotine Alliance*. Their brief is to promote '…ways of reducing harm from cigarette smoking without necessarily giving up the use of nicotine.'

According to their website[54], of the current eight members of the Board of Trustees, only two seem to have any scientific or medical credentials. One is Gerry Stimson, a public health sociologist (whatever that is) who enthuses that e-cigarettes 'can deliver a satisfying hit of nicotine and also emulate some of the rituals and behaviours associated with smoking, making them more appealing.'[55] The other is Paddy Costall who, interestingly, has been involved in substance misuse treatment services. The

---

[53] BMJ 2015;351:h5010
[54] http://nnalliance.org/about-us/board (Accessed September 2015.)
[55] http://blogs.bmj.com/bmj/2013/10/03/gerry-stimson-a-life-or-death-moment-for-tobacco-policy

E-Cigarette Circus

rest are former smokers, now turned to vaping since a number of years, who seem terrified their new-found allegedly safe way of continuing to be addicted to the poison nicotine will be undermined by proposed legislation to regulate e-cigarettes as medicines. They want e-cigs with their myriad forms and flavours on open sale so they can continue to poison themselves with nicotine without the harm of smoking cigarettes.

Another trustee, Dave Dorn, sporting three gold rings and a necklace, who admits to being a vaper of five years standing having for the previous forty-three years smoked sixty cigarettes a day, says vaping is a lifestyle choice and compares it to a child's protective gear for skateboarding.[56]

Does he get comparable fun by sucking vapourised nicotine into his lungs? At any rate, he says (paraphrasing slightly) it's 'sexy, pleasant, enjoyable, nice.' Is it, indeed. Or is it the relief of the temporary discomfort of the withdrawal symptoms of the poison nicotine provided by the previous vaping session which is perceived as sexy, pleasant, etc.?

You can sense the panic at the prospect of e-cigarettes being regulated in the comments of trustee Allan Beard:

> A lifelong heavy smoker from 14 until 59 years of age, I discovered vaping in February 2013 after a little research, and completely switched away from tobacco cigarettes within days. Bewildered and bemused that upon discovery and conversion to a far safer alternative I found there were efforts from many quarters to regulate e-cigarettes out of existence.

What about the completely safe alternative of not using the poison nicotine at all?

It's unfortunate that this prospect seems beyond contemplation for the long list of supporters of the *Alliance*. You only need to

---

[56] https://www.youtube.com/watch?v=RndxxV2cvN4 (Accessed September 2015.)

read their comments on the website to see most of them are hooked on the poison nicotine delivered via e-cigs. Their plaint boils down to this: if e-cigs are allegedly harmless to the user and bystanders what's the objection to them being on sale to adults? The objections are as follows:

- This is a huge, unregulated, public-health experiment. It surely can't do you any good to inhale into your lungs vapourised nicotine together with flavourings, the carcinogen formaldehyde, glycerin and glycol ethers, preservatives etc., many times a day, every day, for years or even decades. There's no need to do this. Why take the risk?
- Common sense tells you children and young people will take up e-cigarettes and some will try smoking as well, when they otherwise wouldn't. (See footnote 47, and there are plenty of other studies.)
- It's an illusion that vaping of itself is enjoyable. But because of this widespread misperception, it's likely many people will try it and become hooked.
- Does it help smokers quit? Possibly, but then it should be used in a regulated way for this purpose only. It's defeatist to swap one way of being addicted to the poison nicotine for another, even if e-cigarettes are supposedly less harmful than smoking.
- Most of these objections to e-cigarettes could be set aside if, as already mentioned, *conventional cigarettes were banned at the same time* that e-cigarettes are allowed on open sale – but can you see that happening?

The e-cigarette industry is already generating huge profits and cigarette companies are at the forefront of this trend. E-cigarettes are now a billion dollar industry in the USA.[57] If one looks at the history of how tobacco companies have perpetrated the biggest confidence trick in the history of the world by falsely promoting smoking as a way to achieve sophistication, sexual attractiveness, relaxation, freshness and – incredibly – good health[58], it's clear they're not going to pass up this opportunity of even vaster profits.

---

[57] Elliott SE. Cigarette Makers' Ads Echo Tobacco's Heyday. N Y Times Web 29 August 2013. http://www.nytimes.com/2013/08/30/business/media/e-cigarette-makers-ads-echo-tobaccos-heyday.html

[58] Proctor, Robert N. *Golden Holocaust: Origins of the Cigarette Catastrophe and the Case for Abolition.* University of California Press, 2011.

Chapter 17

Highly Esteemed Organ

Further examples of the rarefied region which the 'tobacco control community' inhabits can be found in the previously mentioned highly esteemed organ calling itself, indeed, *Tobacco Control*. One article from America deals with *Public education about the relative harm of tobacco products: an intervention for tobacco control professionals.*[59]

Now here's an idea to ponder. Tobacco control professionals. Who could these be? Professional, as opposed the amateur sort, of people who seek to 'control' tobacco? It conjures an image of men with canisters of weed killer on their backs roaming the lanes and fields and spraying tobacco plants wherever they may be found. (I understand that an excellent weed killer can be made from the liquid obtained by boiling tobacco.) It also brings to mind the image of the men in green uniforms who patrol certain streets in Tokyo and other cities in Japan, and when they come upon a smoker, politely draw his or her attention to the ordinance which prohibits smoking while walking and proffer a portable ash-tray or impose a fine.

Unfortunately, in the sense in which it is used in the article, many tobacco control professionals don't seem very professional, because they don't even know that cigarette smoking is more harmful than using smokeless tobacco. The conclusion is that:

> *Public education campaigns are urgently needed for tobacco control professionals and consumers to increase awareness and understanding of the continuum of risk among tobacco products.*

---

[59] Beiner L, Nyman AL, Stapanov I, *et al. Tob Control* 2014;23:385-388.

The meaning of this badly written sentence is elusive, but I guess the authors are trying to say they think there is an urgent need for tobacco control professionals (whatever these may be) to be better informed about the relative risks of different consumer products which enable you to poison yourself with nicotine.

This is typical of the muddled thinking of people who write learned articles for the afore-mentioned scholarly journal. It's impossible to rank with any certainty the safety of different nicotine delivery devices except in broad terms such as that smokeless tobacco is less harmful than smoked tobacco and that e-cigarettes are (probably) less harmful still. But they are all harmful! Nonetheless, is the expectation that if nicotine delivery devices *could* be ranked in order of decreasing harmfulness, everyone would want to use the one at the bottom of the list?

In the same edition of this journal there is another offering, also from America, with the long-winded title: *Electronic nicotine delivery system (electronic cigarette) awareness, use, reactions and beliefs: a systematic review.*[60]

A systematic review is a study of work by other researchers. The papers are selected according to certain criteria, such as that they are written in English and are of a high scientific standard, etc.

These researchers considered 244 papers and settled on forty-nine which met their criteria. To save having to write out repeatedly the term 'electronic nicotine delivery systems', meaning electronic cigarettes or e-cigarettes, they used the acronym ENDS. (There's an inconsistency with singular and plural: in the title it's 'system', but in the text it's 'systems', which in a sense is just as well otherwise the acronym would have to be ENDSs.) The stated object was to review the literature, but the paper seems to have been written as an *end* in itself and is full of the all-too-common lazy writing which such acronyms encourage:

---

[60] Pepper JK, Brewer NT. *Tob Control* 2014;23:375-384

Smoking is a Psychological Problem

The majority of ENDS users believe that ENDS can help people quit or reduce smoking and they often use ENDS themselves for this reason.

So this paper, which runs to nearly eight pages, will be able to be added to the list of the ninety-two references they cite, thus increasing the already voluminous literature on the subject. That aside, let's see what insights are to be found in the article.

It notes (twice) that e-cigarettes are controversial and they point out that in addition to liquid nicotine they contain four major tobacco-specific nitrosamines (cancer-causing chemicals) and propylene glycol (used in anti-freeze and many other products). I can't think it will do you any good to inhale that stuff into your lungs many times a day, every day for years on end.

Let's skip to the conclusion. The authors muse:

If we better understand why ENDS may be attractive to some vulnerable populations (eg, teenagers think ENDS are fashionable), we can craft and deliver effective messages that deter use.

Oh, such wisdom! Of course impressionable teenagers may think e-cigarettes are fashionable. But if they can craft and deliver effective messages (they wouldn't want to craft and deliver ineffective messages, would they) they might be able to deter use!

I can tell them how to deter use. Ban them. We don't need another nicotine delivery device. Otherwise you have a ludicrous situation where these products are on sale but people are urged not to buy them.

Was there *any* point in writing this article? The authors themselves seem to have had doubts because they say:

...because the quality of the studies included in this review varies tremendously, readers should interpret the findings with care.

Oh dear. Then they repeat:

> *In sum, concerns about ENDS include their safety, lack of regulation, possibility of gateway use* (may encourage people to smoke cigarettes who otherwise wouldn't) *and potential for dual use* (smoking cigarettes and using e-cigarettes) *or avoidance of existing smoking restrictions.*

Next, they go on to note:

> *...the possibility that ENDS could prove to be a valuable harm reduction tool for addicted adult smokers...*

You don't need a 'tool' to reduce harm from smoking. You just need to stop smoking! As for addicted adult smokers, are there any other kinds?

The paper *ends* on a whimper:

> *...as we learn more about the safety of ENDS and their efficacy as a quit tool, we will hopefully be able to design better tobacco control and cessation programmes in the future.*

Good luck.

Chapter 18

Waterpipes in Wonderland

Do you remember the charming children's book *Alice in Wonderland* and the scene with the supercilious hookah-smoking caterpillar? Now hookahs, also known as shishas, nargiles or waterpipes are back in the news. The fantasy quality of the medical perspective on waterpipes is shown in yet another editorial in *The British Medical Journal*, written by a certain Professor Wasim Maziak.[61]

The piece is entitled: *Rise of Waterpipe Smoking*. But the subtitle is: *A global public health epidemic in need of a clear and comprehensive regulatory approach.* Does he mean there is an epidemic of public health? That wouldn't be a bad thing. Oh, I see – he's trying to say: 'The global waterpipe epidemic needs regulation.' (He wouldn't call for an unclear or non-comprehensive regulatory approach, would he.) Apart from that, there seems to be an epidemic of the use of the word global in his writing, for example:

> ...waterpipes' popularity among youth took off, first in the Middle East, and soon globally. How could a "cultural" habit become such a global phenomenon in record time?... Simultaneously, the burgeoning global economy and advancements in communication and social networking helped propel waterpipes onto the global stage...

What are waterpipes? Professor Maziak tells us:

> The waterpipe...is a centuries old method of tobacco use that has its roots in Eastern societies. In its most common

---
[61] BMJ 2015;350:h1991

form, charcoal heated air is passed through a tobacco mixture to produce smoke, which is bubbled through water before inhalation by the smoker.

But he cautions:

The mistaken belief that smoke is "filtered" as it passes through water accounts for the misperception of waterpipes as benign compared with cigarettes...

It gets worse:

Studies clearly show waterpipe smokers' exposure to nicotine, toxicants, and carcinogens are associated with smoking-induced disease. In fact, exposure to some toxicants such as carbon monoxide and heavy metals is so high that unique health problems may result.

He makes a further comment on the problems of these devices, but doesn't seem to appreciate its significance:

As the waterpipe is increasingly providing youth with their first experience of tobacco, those who become waterpipe dependent are likely to resort to the more accessible cigarettes **to deal with their urges.** (Emphasis added.)

It's important to note that those who become waterpipe dependent (i.e., nicotine dependent), need somehow to deal with *urges*. That is, urges to *keep putting nicotine into their bodies*. And why do they need to do that, when they didn't before they started using waterpipes? The reader by now will have no difficulty in understanding that it's because they're suffering from the temporary discomfort of withdrawal symptoms of the nicotine they dosed themselves with a little while previously with the waterpipe, which they experience as an urge to do it again – and again and again and again.

What to do about it? Professor Maziak's view (with my comments in parenthesis):

> *Major tobacco regulatory initiatives should include waterpipe specific policies* (groan) *such as bans on flavouring, clean indoor air policies* (whatever that means) *for waterpipe venues, age limits on smoking in café settings* (why not say cafés instead of café settings?) *and requiring large health warnings on waterpipes...*

We're clearly in Wonderland but instead of the magic bottle labelled 'Drink me', we have a waterpipe, legally available to adults only, with unflavoured tobacco, in a café setting with a clean-air policy and a large health warning saying 'Don't smoke me!' Lewis Carroll would have been proud.

What the good Professor doesn't seem to realise is that waterpipes, like all types of nicotine delivery devices, don't need to be regulated. They need to be banned.

Chapter 19

Cigars Are OK – Or Are They?

Just in case anyone thinks cigars are more benign than cigarettes, let's listen to Boris Johnson, mayor of London:

> *Years ago my wife and I had a baby, and I was so elated I went out into I think it was Highbury Fields it was the middle of winter I had a cigar and I sort of think I wasn't doing any harm to anybody else.*[62]

Ah, but he is now. He's perpetuating the idea that smoking a cigar is something you do when you want to celebrate. People may be influenced by what this colourful high profile figure says and think smoking a celebratory cigar is OK – and nothing to do with smoking cigarettes.

The curious idea that cigars are something special also emerges periodically from the pages of the British coffee-table magazine *Country Life*. For example, in a recent edition there was an article by their cigar correspondent (yes, they do have such an one) who goes by the name of Bolivar. He mentions the venerable designer and 'greatest living English cigar smoker' (*sic*), Sir Terence Conran. There is Sir Terence in the photo, impeccably attired, standing in a garden, his pleasant face beaming up at us while he expertly clutches a fat cigar in his right hand. However, the mention of Sir Terence is only to introduce a cigar known as Epicure No. 2 which had this effect on Bolivar when he smoked it:

---

[62] *Daily Mail* online 24 October 2014

Smoking is a Psychological Problem

> *I was prepared for a bit of a headache when I set fire to it and, by the time I reached the end, I needed to sit down.*[63]

The illusion of the wonders of cigar smoking is further demonstrated in the link in this article to a video called *How to smoke a cigar*, featuring Edward Sahakian, the proprietor of the cigar shop Davidoff of London.

To the accompaniment of a Vivaldi concerto to set the mood, Mr Sahakian tells us, in his mildly laryngitic voice (paraphrasing slightly):

> *My first cigar starts as part of my breakfast...It's very important to choose the right cigar for the occasion... this morning, as I've had a nice breakfast, and a coffee, to complement that I'm going to smoke one of favourite cigars... it's a mild cigar, smooth, it will probably keep me going for a good hour, an hour and a half... and sometimes I could stretch that into a couple of hours...Before I do anything with the cigar I always look at it. It's very important (coughs)...it's the love affair (smiles), the first sight...*[64]

So he's had a nice breakfast, and a coffee, and there may be Vivaldi in the background, and he's set up for the day. Indeed, I often start the day myself in this way. But what does Mr Sahakian do then? Over the next hour, hour-and-a-half or even two hours he proceeds to absorb through the lining of his mouth into his bloodstream nicotine and many other poisonous chemicals. And this, it seems, is a love affair!

Will somebody please tell me: are we non-cigar smokers missing something?

---

[63] *Country Life*, 29 January 2014, p89
[64] http://www.youtube.com/watch?v=UnSNJf5cnhs

Chapter 20

Plain Packaging

The government claims that by legislating to require plain packaging of cigarettes they're trying to discourage children from starting to smoke. (I suppose they mean standard packaging, because the proposed plain packs are anything but, being adorned with a variety of horrible pictures of the sort of things one might see in a pathology museum.) Fine, but it's rather a roundabout way of doing this. It's as if they're saying to the public, 'Don't buy this, it's dangerous.' Or are they trying to put people off buying cigarettes altogether? Then why not say so? If this is the case, the logical step would be to start the process of banning tobacco sales.

I'm no friend of the tobacco companies, but it seems to me they have a point in that their right to display their brand images on the packages of their poisonous (but legal) products will be infringed. Already a large proportion of the pack is taken up with health warnings and horrible pictures. Now it's proposed that nearly all of the pack will be taken up with health warnings and horrible pictures and the name of the maker will be relegated to standard small type at the bottom of the front and at the underside of the pack. The background colour is described as 'Pantone 448C (a drab dark brown)' but which I think could more accurately be called cow-shit green. So now, instead of smokers buying a pack of, say, Marlboro, L&M or Lucky Strike, they will be choosing between 'damages teeth and gums', 'causes peripheral vascular disease', 'causes blindness', etc.

There's a video put out by Cancer Research UK[65] to promote plain packaging. It shows children, who appear to be aged

---

[65] https://www.youtube.com/watch?v=c_z-4S8iicc (viewed 17 March 2015)

between about seven and eleven, who are given empty cigarette packs to handle and comment on how they appear to them. This is a selection of what they say:

- I like this one because it's got red in it and red is my favourite colour
- It reminds me of a Ferrari
- It looks kind of like the sun
- Is that a royal sign? It looks quite posh
- It's really bright colours and it would be quite fun to play with and it makes you happy just by looking at it
- This one is actually quite pretty – Yeah, pink, pink, pink
- The pictures actually look quite nice, like ice-cubes and mint
- It makes you feel you're in a wonderland of happiness

The film ends with the written statement:

Unbranding cigarette packs won't stop everyone from smoking, but it will give millions of kids one less reason to start.

Apart from the dubious ethics of allowing these children to handle attractive cigarette packs – might it not encourage them to smoke if the hypothesis of the film is correct? – it seems to me this whole campaign for standard packaging is a distraction from the real issue. Again, something is being done: the government is bringing in legislation to 'protect our kids' by making cigarette packs less attractive. Two cheers for the government.

Is the push to plain packaging based on the kind of research mentioned above? If so, it seems mightily unscientific to me. Do children start smoking because they see an attractive cigarette pack in a shop, even if it's on the top shelf, and say, 'Ooh, look at that, it's like a Ferrari, it's red – my favourite colour! I must try smoking!' Or do they say, contemplating another pack, 'I think

I'll try smoking – that pack makes me feel I'll be in a wonderland of happiness!' Do they? I submit that they don't. Children want to smoke because they see *other people* smoking and wish to imitate it. So they have already decided to obtain cigarettes somehow. Do they then look at the pack, note with disgust and loathing the horrible pictures – and change their minds? Where is the evidence for that? I think it will do little to put children off. They might even be *more* tempted to do it to try to appear grown-up enough *not* be put off by the horrible pictures.

Whatever the packs looks like, why aren't children put off by their first experiences of smoking? When I ask my smoker patients to describe the effects of the first experimental cigarette they tried behind the bicycle shed aged twelve or fifteen, they usually have no difficulty in recalling them, even decades later. They say things like:

- It wasn't pleasant
- It made me cough and I felt dizzy
- It was horrible. I felt sick and had to lie down

But that didn't put them off – they were hooked from the first puff!

First it was the big debate about passive smoking: was it or wasn't it harmful? Then it was the banning of smoking in public indoor areas: would it put pubs and restaurants out of business? Now it's e-cigarettes and plain packaging.

It seems to me all these debates are nothing more than delaying tactics. Big Tobacco will argue and wheedle and lobby and engage expensive lawyers and pay for independent grass roots campaigns and for completely unbiased scientists to do studies to show (amazing!) that passive smoking is not harmful, pubs and restaurants will go out of business, plain packaging will not work and anyhow is unnecessary because (would you believe it!) Big Tobacco does not target children and it will encourage cigarettes smuggling (very wicked! – and what good corporate citizens the tobacco companies are to wish to uphold the law). All of this is obfuscation and a distraction from the real issue. While the pseudo-debate goes on about the desirability and effectiveness of plain packaging, what does Big Tobacco do in the meantime – the meantime being measured in years and even decades?

It goes merrily on making and selling cigarettes.

Also in the meantime, the medical profession is getting really exercised over plain packaging. *The British Medical Journal* in June 2014 published an open letter[66] with the heading *Government must draw up law on tobacco plain packaging soon*. It was signed by eminent chest specialists and experts in public health and epidemiology and by 584 others. After reminding readers that

> *Smoking related disease remains the main cause of preventable deaths in the UK, killing more than 100,000 people each year*

they went on to say

> *Most smokers start in childhood, and exposure to tobacco marketing is known to increase this risk.*

Really? It's supposition masquerading as fact. In support of this statement they cite a 126 page document produced by the University of Stirling called *Plain Packaging: A Systematic Review*. The problem with this review is that it deals only with opinions of the impact of plain packaging and the authors themselves say their conclusions are speculative.

The first paragraph of the letter ends with this remarkable statement:

---

[66] BMJ 2014;348:g3779

Plain Packaging

> *To protect public health, particularly the health of children at risk of becoming smokers, it is therefore necessary and logical to end the marketing of cigarettes and tobacco products*

Except the sentence doesn't end there, as in my view it should. It ends like this:

> *...it is therefore necessary and logical to end the marketing of cigarettes and tobacco products through packaging.*

This verbose sentence is ambiguous. Tobacco products include cigarettes so the word cigarettes could be omitted. Now, do the writers mean that the introduction of plain packaging will bring about the end of the marketing of tobacco products? Is that their wish? Then they should say so clearly. Or do they merely mean to say it's necessary and logical to end that part of the marketing of tobacco products which is done through the current packaging designs? In this case, what is the evidence that the branded packs on sale everywhere (except in Australia) *themselves* contribute to the marketing of tobacco products and thus the uptake of smoking by children? The apposite question is whether the adoption of plain packs will *of itself* result in a decrease in the prevalence of smoking. The answer is unknown and we shall have to await the result of this experiment in Australia.

If it's part of a policy to squeeze the tobacco companies out of existence, that's fine by me, but it should be explicitly stated. Why are governments so afraid of upsetting Big Tobacco? Is it something to do with their huge profits from tobacco tax revenues? If so, this is conflicted and immoral. The extreme of this situation is seen in Japan where the government is required by law to own at least one third of Japan Tobacco's stock.

The evidence cited in support of the claimed necessity of ending the marketing of tobacco products through packaging (whichever way you take it), is a paper in the learned journal *Thorax*[67] of which the first named author is an eminent chest specialist, Nicholas S Hopkinson, who happens also to be the first-named signatory of the open letter.

So he's quoting his own work, saying:

> *There is compelling evidence that young people are susceptible to branding and advertising and are influenced by the depiction of smoking in films.*

Wait a minute. The letter is about branding of the packages, not smoking depicted in films. Anyway, in support of this statement he cites two other papers, one of which only deals with films[68], so we needn't consider it further.

The other citation[69] does indeed deal with cigarette packs. It's a study that involved exposing adolescents to cigarette packs and eliciting their comments. The results, not surprisingly, showed:

> *When brand elements such as color, branded fonts, and imagery were progressively removed from cigarette packs, adolescents perceived packs to be less appealing, rated attributes of a typical smoker of the pack less positively, and had more negative expectations of cigarette taste.*

So they proved the obvious, but what has this got to do with young people in the real world? It's like the Cancer Research UK video mentioned above. But do unattractive packs mean children will be less inclined to start smoking? We don't know, but I suspect any effect will be marginal, considering why children start smoking in the first place. Or it may be hard to judge because it will be compounded by other factors such as increased prices

---

[67] doi:10.1136/thoraxjnl-2013-204379
[68] *Thorax* 2011;66:875-83
[69] *Journal of Adolescent Health* 2010;46:385–92

of cigarettes – which does seem to work in reducing smoking prevalence. Therefore, it's an assumption for Dr Hopkinson to claim, as he appears to do, that introducing plain packaging will result in fewer children smoking.

It's difficult to understand why such an almost hysterical letter with its huge number of signatories was written, and why *The British Medical Journal* published it. If plain packaging were introduced that would solve the smoking problem? It seems to me that such an ill-judged outcry (ill-judged because it's likely to be ineffective) arose, once again, *because of a lack of understanding about why people start smoking, why they continue and why they find it so difficult to stop.*

I suggest they should have written, instead, an open letter to the government along the following lines:

> 'Smoking-related disease remains the main cause of preventable deaths in the UK, killing more than 100,000 people each year.
>
> To protect public health, particularly the health of children at risk of becoming smokers, it is therefore necessary and logical to institute legislation to ban the production and sale of tobacco products.
>
> Yours, &c.'

PART THREE

Research

Chapter 21

Smoking Research

Why is so much research being done on smoking? Apart from scientific curiosity, grants are awarded, learned papers published, conferences convened and opinions sought from those eminent in the field by governments and the media. And careers have even been built on it.

Let's look at some typical research. At the University College of San Francisco there's a department called the Center for Tobacco Control Research and Education. Quite a mouthful of a name. They carried out a study entitled *Pharmacologic Basis of Racial Difference in Nicotine Dependence*.[70] The lead author was Neal Benowitz, Professor of Medicine, Bioengineering and Therapeutic Sciences. He concluded, hypothetically, that:

> ...there are racial differences in metabolism that may explain different patterns of smoking, and that this in turn influences the reasons why smokers continue to self-administer nicotine (i.e., continue to smoke).

Fascinating stuff, no doubt, but what practical use is it? It seems to me the answer is none.

Whatever sort of smoker you are or whatever race you happen to come from, the way to overcome the problem is the same for all: STOP SMOKING.

From the scientific point of view, a lot of research is being done to try to understand the mechanisms of addiction: what

---

[70] https://tobacco.ucsf.edu/pharmacologic-basis-racial-difference-nicotine-dependence

neurotransmitters and other brain activities are involved, whether there is a genetic component that makes some people more likely than others to smoke, etc. And the reason for doing this, it seems, is the fond hope that, maybe, one day, more specific 'interventions' will be devised which will be more effective in helping smokers to quit.

I submit that, interesting though all this research may be, in practical terms it's pointless. Enough is already known. It can be summarised as follows:

1. Smoking causes cancer and numerous other nasty diseases.
2. People smoke only because of addiction to nicotine.
3. The cure for this is to stop smoking.
4. When they have stopped they must want to stay stopped.
5. Young people should not start smoking.

Reason 1 is indisputable. Even the tobacco companies admit it.

However, we now start running into difficulties. By no means all so-called experts are agreed on 2. They think the reason people smoke is due *in addition* to other disparate but important factors, for example, chemical or structural changes in the brain.[71][72] It is also widely believed that people smoke because of 'cues' or the routines associated with smoking, such as when having a drink, or after a meal or when talking on the phone. Some other reasons which seem rather far-fetched are also mentioned: poverty[73], or because of a perceived lack of support to stop smoking.

Point 3 is where it gets interesting. It's at the heart of the problem. For a start, most smokers don't *really* want to quit, at least not right now. Are there any interventions which could make smokers *want* to quit? For something so hazardous to health as cigarette smoking it's absurd it's allowed at all. I have actually had smokers tell me

---

[71] *Neuropsychopharmacology* (2014) **39**, 1816–1822; doi:10.1038/npp.2014.48
[72] Chaloupka FJ, et al. Tob Control 2015;24:115
[73] Hausten KO. Eur J Cardiovasc Prev Rehabil. 2006 Jun;13(3):312-8

they don't believe the health warnings because, they say, if it's true cigarettes are dangerous they wouldn't be allowed.

As for horrible pictures and health warnings, how about this:

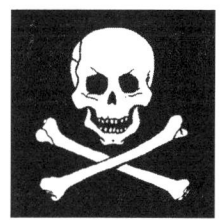

DANGER!
CIGARETTE SMOKE IS POISONOUS
IF YOU SMOKE IT MAY KILL YOU
YOU HAVE BEEN WARNED
DON'T DO IT!
THROW THESE CIGARETTES AWAY
STOP SMOKING TODAY

Something similar has already been tried, although with a different aim. In 1991 an entrepreneur by the name of B J Cunningham established The Enlightened Tobacco Company which sold cigarettes called 'Death' featuring a skull and crossbones on the pack. The company flopped.

In Tobacco Control Industry-speak this would be called a Graphic Warning Label.

In spite of the failure of Mr Cunningham's company, it's obvious, I would have thought, that if you show repulsive pictures on most of the surface of cigarette packs this may produce aversion or even fear in potential customers. Presumably this is why such pictures are put on the packs. However, in the Tobacco Control Industry world, common sense is not enough; they need to *prove* it. And one way to do this, would you believe it, is through what is known as functional magnetic resonance imaging (fMRI) of the brain.

This is a technique of showing on a screen which parts of the brain use more oxygen during certain activities, such as performing mental arithmetic or, indeed, viewing horrible pictures. It's a brilliant invention with all sorts of potential applications. However, at present our knowledge of how the brain works is in its infancy and fMRI is a fairly crude and indirect way of seeing what's going on.

Nonetheless, an intrepid group of four researchers from the University of Pennsylvania and a psychiatrist from Harvard Medical School recruited twenty-four smokers as guinea pigs.[74] They subjected them to fMRI to try to see what happened in their brains when they experienced an emotional reaction (ER) while viewing graphic warning labels (GWLs) of pictures of cancers which smoking can induce. (Many medical papers are littered with non-standard abbreviations of this sort.)

The earth-shattering, albeit circular, conclusion of all this work?

> ...the higher ER GWLs produced a greater reduction in the craving to smoke...these findings provide further support for the idea that it is the strong emotional response that drives the behavioural impact from GWLs.

To put it simply: horrible pictures on cigarette packs may put people off smoking.

Instead of leaving it at that, however, such conclusions are always regarded as tentative and indicating a need for more research, so the industry is self-perpetuating. They continue:

> These results suggest that the ER elicited by graphic labels contributes to their behavioural impact. Controlled longitudinal studies are required to determine whether our

---

[74] Doi:10.1136/tobaccocontrol-2014-051993

findings are maintained over time and translate from the cognitive, neurophysiological correlates of effectiveness to the clinical outcomes.

In plain English: do horrible pictures on cigarette packs put people off smoking?

I have often wondered whether those working in the Tobacco Control Industry live in ivory towers. Now I know this is wrong – they live on a different planet.

Chapter 22

Futile Smoking Research

One can take almost any article in the medical literature on smoking research to see the futility of much of the current work in this field.

For example, *The British Medical Journal* recently published a 'State of the Art Review' entitled *Smoking cessation and reduction in people with chronic mental illness*[75], which

> ...critically assesses the effectiveness of smoking cessation treatments for people with schizophrenia, unipolar and bipolar depression, anxiety disorders, and post-traumatic stress disorder.

This opening sentence makes two dubious assumptions: that smoking cessation is something that needs treatment, and that there's something special about smokers who have been diagnosed as suffering from a mental illness.

The possible connection between smoking and mental illness is derived, it seems, from trawling the literature and coming upon a paper in a scholarly journal called *Psychological Bulletin*. In this paper the authors discuss an idea they have thought up about a connection between anxiety, depression and smoking. Or at least I think that's what they're trying to do. But if we read no further than the abstract, we find this[76] – I promise I'm not making it up:

> We propose that transdiagnostic emotional vulnerabilities-core biobehavioral traits reflecting maladaptive responses to

---

[75] BMJ 2015;351:h4065
[76] doi: 10.1037/bul0000003

emotional states that underpin multiple types of emotional psychopathology-link various anxiety and depressive psychopathologies to smoking. (sic)

It's not even a proper sentence. No matter how you struggle with it (and why should you have to struggle?) this careless writing is meaningless nonsense.

Endless attempts of this sort by workers in the Tobacco Control Industry to try and find different 'interventions' for supposedly different types of smokers, whether they are so-called hardcore[77], pregnant[78], prisoners[79], or – the latest category – mental cases, in all the research it generates is like a dog trying to catch its tail. It reminds me of the joke about experiments on rats mentioned in Chapter 16, which could be paraphrased thus: the cigarette is an artefact which, when smoked, produces a paper.

All smokers – whatever their circumstances and irrespective of whether they've been labelled with a medical diagnosis – have the same problem: addiction to the poison nicotine. And the solution is the same for all of them: stop smoking.

Although it may have a fatal outcome, smoking itself is not a disease for which treatment is needed, and it's counter-productive to regard it in this way – because smokers are thereby reinforced in their belief that it's terribly difficult to stop without medical help.

The poor smoker is in a dilemma. She knows it's hazardous to health and wants to stop for this obvious reason; but on the other hand she doesn't *really* want to stop because of a perception that smoking is enjoyable or helpful, or both. Nonetheless, suppose she decides to make the effort to quit. How to go about it? Even this question is odd. There's no method or way or treatment you need to follow. You just stop! But because of all the publicity about nicotine maintenance products and stop-smoking medicines and

---

[77] BMJ 2003;326:0-c
[78] BMJ 2014;348:g1808
[79] BMJ2014;349:g4946

Smoking is a Psychological Problem

now e-cigarettes, to say nothing of specialist smoking cessation clinics, you could be forgiven for thinking it's very hard to stop on your own – in spite of evidence to the contrary cited in Chapter 9.

If you take the plunge and try the orthodox approach, to start with you will have it drummed into you how difficult it will be – look at the NHS Stoptober and Smokefree campaigns. They tell you all the horrible withdrawal symptoms and 'cravings' you are likely to suffer and they may even measure the carbon monoxide in your breath. Then, very likely you'll be offered a nicotine product – when you're trying to get off nicotine! – or a drug to cause a chemical imbalance in your brain[80] to counteract the drugged state you're already in because of your smoking.

Whereas it's a reasonable supposition that drugs used in mental illness can only work (if they work at all) by disturbing brain chemistry, it's another matter entirely to say chemical imbalances in the brain are the *cause* of mental illnesses. Yet this is what the State of the Art Review implies:

> *Depression is associated with low resting levels of intrasynaptic dopamine, and smokers experience larger increases in striatal dopamine after smoking a cigarette than those without a history of depression.*

Three references from the 1990s are cited in support of this statement: they are to studies of a technique called positron emission tomography (similar to fMRI mentioned in the previous chapter). This produces images indicating blood flow in various regions of the brain, but it's not the same thing as showing the actual levels of dopamine. In recognition of this, the results of the cited studies are reported cautiously, in terms such as: 'These findings support the theory that smokers with depression have

---

[80] Gøtzsche P. *Deadly Medicines and Organized Crime: How big pharma has corrupted healthcare.* 2013

Futile Smoking Research

abnormal dopamine function' and 'These data could indicate an increase of dopamine receptor density in depression.' There's no justification for treating a theory as if it's a proven fact. It's impossible at present to measure levels of dopamine or serotonin or any other chemical transmitter in the living human brain, so it's merely fanciful to say an increase in dopamine occurs after smoking a cigarette. And even if it's true, what then? This underwhelming conclusion:

> *The research reviewed here indicates that smokers with chronic mental illness can quit with standard cessation approaches...*

They might have saved themselves the bother.

Chapter 23

The Road to Hell

There's a well-known proverb: the road to hell is paved with good intentions.

These days virtually all smokers know smoking is hazardous to health and a waste of money – at least if they pause to think about it. Every time they light up they wish they weren't doing it, but for some reason seem unable to desist.

It matters not one jot or tittle whether smokers *intend* to stop smoking. What matters is whether they *actually* stop permanently – or not. Since smokers are probably secretly ashamed of their smoking, if asked in surveys if they intend to quit, they may indeed say, Yes, they intend to quit. And some of them may well go on to attempt to quit, and of those who make such attempts, a certain proportion will manage to stop. Incidentally, what does it mean when someone says they are 'trying' to stop? It's an excuse smokers use as a justification to carry on smoking, the 'Yes, but' response, and often emerges if someone is asked whether they smoke: 'Yes, but I'm trying to quit.'

So, what is the point of doing research to find out what motivates smokers to say they intend to quit, whether such intentions result in quit attempts and whether such attempts succeed?

Even if it means scraping the barrel, some workers in the Tobacco Control Industry apparently *do* seem to find a point in this sort of study. No doubt they need to justify their salaries and the funding they receive as well as gaining prestige by having learned papers published in scholarly journals. Or scholarly papers published in learned journals.

And what about the funding? For example, the result of the combined efforts of eight researchers from four countries was a paper entitled *Smoking-related thoughts and microbehaviours* (sic), *and their predictive power for quitting.*[81] This was supported by grants from no less than nine prestigious bodies[82] who presumably were persuaded that this was pretty important work. The total must have amounted to a tidy sum. But how much? I wrote to the lead investigator, Dr Lin Li of the Cancer Council Victoria, Australia, and asked him. He refused to tell me.

The main object of this paper was to examine these smoking-related thoughts and microbehaviors among Chinese smokers, though only one of the authors was based in China.

Looking at it a little more closely I can perhaps see why Dr Li is so coy about the grant money he received. Maybe it's because the paper is a laugh a minute – except there's nothing funny about smoking. Let's start with the first sentence of the Introduction:

> *Negative attitudes to smoking reliably predict intentions to quit smoking and quitting behaviours.*

Prediction of intentions to quit – I ask you! We're back on the road to hell. And by the way, what's the difference between quitting and quitting behaviours?

As if this idea hasn't been flogged to death, it's resurrected by their reference to studies of:

> *...microbehaviours that result from negative thoughts, such as forgoing a cigarette or butting out a cigarette before it is finished are also associated with increased subsequent likelihood of quitting...we refer to frequency of such thoughts*

---

[81] Doi:10.1136/tobaccocontrol-2013-051384

[82] US National Cancer Institute at the National Institutes of Health, Roswell Park Transdisciplinary Tobacco Use Research Center, Robert Wood Johnson Foundation, Canadian Institutes for Health Research, National Health and Medical Research Council of Australia, Cancer Research UK, Chinese Center for Disease Control and Prevention, Ontario Institute for Cancer Research and Canadian Cancer Society Research Institute.

and microbehaviours collectively as 'microindicators of concern about smoking'...[which] appear to be reliably associated with subsequently making quit attempts [but] their relationships with quit success among those who try, is less clear.

What's so special about putting out a cigarette before it's finished? Smokers often do this – just look a used ash-tray (not a pretty sight). And sticking the word 'micro' onto the front of behaviours and indicators, it seems to me, does nothing to assist comprehension. Anyway, let me try and recast this in plain English:

'If a smoker foregoes a cigarette or puts one out before it is finished this means he or she is concerned about the dangers of smoking and is more likely to quit. However, if smokers have negative attitudes to smoking and are concerned about its effects, they may try to stop but may not succeed.'

All clear?
Further, in case you missed it the first time around, they quote other studies which conclude:

...the frequency of prematurely butting out cigarettes due to noticing cigarette pack warnings was positively associated with subsequent quit attempts, however, it was negatively associated with at least 1 month of sustained abstinence among those who made quit attempts...forgoing cigarettes as a result of noticing health warnings on packs was a consistent prospective predictor of making quit attempts, but had no consistent relationship with maintaining abstinence for at least 1 month. (The word prospective is redundant.)

So, if you're worried about smoking you may try to stop, but if you're frightened by the health warnings on the packs you may try to stop but won't necessarily succeed.

Now what about China? This is a country with a huge smoking problem and where tobacco marketing and use are largely unrestricted. The authors predict that:

> ...*in China there will be less* (sic) *smokers highly motivated to quit but with less capacity to do so.*

And the main overall conclusion (paraphrasing slightly)?

> *In China, unlike in the West, quit attempts were largely unrelated to sustained abstinence. Activities to drive up quitting are likely to be essentially the same as those used successfully in the West.*

So now what?

Instead of all this dry-as-dust research into intentions to quit smoking, the important questions which need to be considered are these:

Why do people start smoking?
Why do they continue?
Why does it seem so difficult to stop?

The answers should be obvious. People start because of *other smokers*, they continue because of *nicotine addiction* and the reason it seems so difficult to stop is because of *nicotine addiction*. In any case, if research is undertaken surely it should be with the ultimate aim of discovering how to reduce smoking prevalence to zero.

The solution to this problem is provided by some real people in China who were interviewed by the BBC soon after the introduction of a law banning smoking in indoor public places in Beijing in June 2015.[83] One says:

> *I think a ban would be hard to enforce in China. There are simply too many smokers.*

Another comments:

> **If you really want to ban smoking then you should shut down the cigarette factories.**

What about doing research into how to do that?

---

[83] http://www.bbc.com/news/world-asia-32954884. Accessed 17 August 2015.

PART FOUR
Big Tobacco

Chapter 24

Big Tobacco and the BBC

If you'd had nothing better to do on two days in May 2014 you might have watched the BBC two-part programme *The Burning Desire* presented by Peter Taylor.[84] He seems to have made a career out of 'investigating smoking and the tobacco industry' and bears more than a passing resemblance to Woody Allen.

In two hours of sound bites Big Tobacco is presented as the bad guy. Its spokesmen say they want to be 'responsible' and readily admit the harm caused by their poisonous products, but they continue to market them, especially in third-world countries with weak or no anti-smoking legislation, and they fight tooth and nail to prevent or delay the introduction of standardised packaging or other measures which might reduce their sales. The good guys (doctors, health ministers, etc.) now hail standardised packaging as a great advance to reduce the attractiveness of cigarettes to young people and thus save lives.

So, what's new?

'Every year more than five million customers of the tobacco industry die' Peter Taylor tells us, and he goes on, 'In this series we investigate how thousands of young people around the world are still taking up smoking every day.' Excuse me? What does he mean *how* young people around the world are still taking up smoking? Obviously, by going into a shop and buying cigarettes or obtaining them from friends and then smoking them. The question should be: *why do governments allow cigarettes to be sold in every corner shop and supermarket?*

Peter Taylor: 'I've spent forty years researching how in the past the industry has dissembled and lied.' *Of course they have*, these 'decent people' (see below).

---

[84] http://www.bbc.co.uk/programmes/b045cjmw

Smoking is a Psychological Problem

Let's hear from the Scientific Director of British American Tobacco (BAT), Dr David O'Reilly. I'll quote him in full:

> So this is a chart which lays out the hundred known toxicants in cigarette smoke. You're inhaling them into your lung and that's why cigarette smoking represents such a risk to health. The carcinogens would be things like benzopyrene, cadmium, lead and mercury. Cigarette smoking is a cause of real and serious diseases. Cancer, particularly cancer of the lung, heart disease, so stroke and heart attack, and respiratory disease such as bronchitis and emphysema, and so for a lifetime smoker about half of them can expect to die prematurely as a result of their cigarette smoking.

This beggars belief. How can he stand there with a straight face and make such an admission? Yet his company still goes on making and selling *billions* of cigarettes. In my opinion, cigarette companies should be indicted for crimes against humanity.

Equally loathsome is another BATman, Kingsley Wheaton:

> I think the future is about tobacco harm reduction. It's about providing a range of alternative nicotine products to consumers. We are indeed the problem. That is **no** reason for us not to be part of the solution...whilst conventional cigarettes will remain the mainstay of our business for a long time...
> (His emphasis.)

Part of the solution, eh? They could be the *whole* of the solution, at least as far as BAT is concerned, by doing the decent thing: STOP MAKING CIGARETTES.

Next we are shown a group of students being interviewed by Peter Taylor on a cold day sitting on a bench outside one of their University buildings. Here are some of their comments:

> *It's horrible coming out in the wind and the weather and everything to have a smoke but you need to do it though, don't you, so…*

> *When you wake up in the morning [smoking] is quite horrible*

> *[Smoking] tastes disgusting when you wake up but…*

In answer to the question why they want a cigarette, they say, speaking together:

> *You need one, Yeah…College is stressful, very stressful, you need 'em more and more*

Then Peter Taylor delivers his *dénouement*: 'The tobacco industry insists it does not target children, but in the UK there's a staggering statistic. Every year 200,000 children aged between eleven and fifteen start smoking.'

On top of this, viewers are reminded that 'When you've got a highly addictive product used by a very large number of people, it's a licence to print money'. Indeed, and that's doubtless why 'BAT manufactures 700 billion (*sic*) cigarettes annually.'

Also featured is Professor Sir Cyril Chantler, a paediatrician who comes over as a rather sweet, naïve man who implores:

> *We have a duty of care to our young people and our children and we should do everything we can to encourage them not to do something which they will regret later in life. I wish the tobacco industry would just accept it. They're decent people, so why don't they just do their very best to help us all to reduce the risk of young people starting to smoke?*

Excuse me a moment while I take out my hanky.
He then goes on to state the obvious:

> *If you can encourage young people not to start [smoking] then you will reduce the suffering and the premature deaths and the huge cost which this imposes to our NHS.*

Too true. But almost everybody is afraid to face up to the glaring paradox: **how can the tobacco industry – which openly admits its products kill six million[85] of its customers worldwide every year – be allowed to carry on making and selling cigarettes?**

It's as if governments are almost powerless towards Big Tobacco, or maybe they just choose a *laissez-faire* attitude. The responsibility is put onto the tobacco companies to admit that their products are harmful, which belatedly they now do, and leave to them to choose to continue to produce and market cigarettes, or not. And in the meantime the best, or perhaps the only, thing to be done is so-called harm reduction, for example, by approving (if not encouraging) 'vaping' – and hope this does indeed prove to be less harmful than smoking.

On standard packaging we hear from James Reilley, the then Irish Health Minister:

> *[Tobacco companies] will argue that we're interfering with intellectual property rights. It would be an extraordinary society that would put the intellectual property rights of multinationals over the right to life of citizens and children particularly. This is a nation that stands on its own two feet and we'll protect our children.*

He is, of course, quite right. But what a strange situation. The way to protect Irish children from being tempted to become nicotine addicts is to put horrible pictures on cigarette packs in the hope it will put them off smoking. Maybe it will work, or maybe it won't.

Peter Taylor sums up:

---

[85] http://www.cancer.org/aboutus/globalhealth/tobacco-control

Big Tobacco and the BBC

> *The tobacco industry [is] going from strength to strength with billion dollar profits and a billion customers worldwide and it seems there's no immediate likelihood of that changing.*

Perhaps for his next programme on smoking and the tobacco industry he might investigate whether this fatalistic conclusion is the only answer to such a scandalous situation.

Chapter 25

Into the Lions' Den

We had a peek at British American Tobacco's UK headquarters in the previous chapter where, among other cynical revelations, their Scientific Director made his well-known but nonetheless shocking admission.

Now let's visit their website, in particular the section called *Discover BAT Science*. Here, you're taken on a conducted tour of their Research & Development laboratories.[86]

We meet an unnamed attractive blonde woman, the Presenter, who starts by telling us:

> *We all know smoking is a cause of serious diseases, including lung cancer, chronic obstructive pulmonary disease and cardiovascular disease. But despite knowing the risks, millions of people still continue to choose to smoke.*

Note the disingenuous juxtaposition of these two sentences: smoking causes serious diseases as we all know, but millions of people continue to choose to smoke.

In other words, if you're a smoker who gets one of these serious diseases, don't blame us – you *knew* it was dangerous but you *continued to choose* to smoke. This tries to hide the fact that people don't continue to choose to smoke. They chose to smoke the first one but thereafter, in spite of knowing the risks, they feel compelled to keep smoking because they became addicted to the poison nicotine.

She goes on:

---

[86] http://www.bat.com/group/sites/uk__9d9kcy.nsf/vwPagesWebLive/DO9P3E5H?opendocument. Accessed 16 August 2015.

I've come to visit British American Tobacco's Research & Development teams to see what they're doing to try to improve their existing products and develop less risky alternatives.

What does she mean BAT is trying to 'improve their existing products'? How can cigarettes be improved? Made less harmful? It's impossible for cigarettes to be made less harmful. The tobacco industry has been pretending to do this for decades, for example by putting ventilation holes in cigarettes so they will give lower tar and nicotine readings on a smoking machine. Then smokers, tricked into thinking such 'light' or 'lite' cigarettes as they were called (it's no longer allowed) were safer, would compensate by covering the ventilation holes or by taking deeper draughts of the poisonous fumes.[87] The only improvement was in the companies' profits.

Not to worry. BAT is also trying to 'develop less risky alternatives'. What good corporate citizens they are!

We are also informed:

What many people don't realise is that it's not nicotine that is the cause of smoking related diseases; it's the smoke itself. Tobacco is a plant and burning it produces smoke which contains six to seven thousand chemicals of which over a hundred are known to be harmful...It's inhaling these toxicants that is the cause of smoking related diseases.

If we take this at its face value, in spite of the contradiction that the poison nicotine itself is by implication safe, then why doesn't BAT just make patches, gum, e-cigarettes and other alternatives to tobacco for putting the poison nicotine into your body, and henceforth STOP MAKING CIGARETTES? I put this

---

[87] Robert N. Proctor, *op. cit.* p372. (No relation of Christopher Proctor mentioned later in this chapter.)

question to their Chief Scientific Officer, Chris Proctor, when I visited their laboratories – see below.

Continuing our tour, attractive blonde Presenter now sporting a white coat, invites us to 'Step inside: explore our biology labs.' What would be going on in there?

> *In the biology department they use a technique called in vitro modelling…that means the study of human cells that are alive but outside the human body…[which] allows the team to study the effect of smoke on diseases like cancer and heart disease.*

Switch to one Katherine Hewett, another scientist who has sold her soul to the BAT devil. By the way, she's not just a common or garden kind of scientist, but a *Bioassessment* Scientist! She cheerfully informs us:

> *This machine replicates the blood flow in the human body and allows the cells to feel at home, and then we add cigarette smoke and the cells become stressed.*

Oh dear. Apart from her patronising way of putting it, the nice warm feeling we have because the cells feel at home in the machine, turns to dismay as we learn that in the presence of cigarette smoke the cells become stressed. Of course they do! Put poison in contact with any living system and observe the damage. Read any medical text-book and it will tell you in no uncertain terms, if patients who smoke suffer heart or lung disease or a host of other illnesses, they should *stop smoking*.

Back to attractive blonde Presenter:

> *So, I hope this has given you a taste of BAT's commitment to developing less risky products. And they're not doing it behind closed doors. They welcome regulators and other*

scientists to visit and they will answer your questions. The only thing hidden away in R&D are world class scientists working on cutting edge technology.

What an utterly breath-taking load of hypocrisy! If these world class scientists, who are working on cutting edge technology, had any decency or integrity they wouldn't be involved with a tobacco company but would put their skills at the service of the sick. The claim of these people to be doing research into developing less harmful delivery devices for the poison nicotine is merely an *excuse* to go on making and selling conventional cigarettes in the meantime – which means a *long* time.

All this investigation into the effects of tobacco smoke on human cell-cultures is just a more sophisticated way of doing the notorious mouse skin-painting tests described in Christopher Proctor's 2003 book, *Sometimes a cigarette is just a cigarette*. Fifty years of this kind of research – and the result? Useless.

In the summer of 2015 I took Doctor Proctor (he has a PhD, not a medical qualification) up on his invitation to visit BAT's headquarters at Southampton in southern England. They kindly provided a taxi for the return journey from London and I accepted their hospitality of a sandwich lunch and coffee.

It was somehow disconcerting passing through the security barrier and into the compound. I had a similar feeling when by coincidence a couple of weeks later I visited the House of the Wannsee Conference outside Berlin, where in 1942 the murder of millions of people was planned by the Nazis. It brought home to me that this is where they do research to manipulate cigarettes for greater profits (£6.1 billion) and to develop new delivery systems for the poison nicotine to be foisted on the public, *in the meantime selling 667 billion cigarettes, worldwide* (2014 figures).[88] In the

---

[88] BMJ 2015;350:h2052

Smoking is a Psychological Problem

UK, where 100,000 people die each year from smoking-related diseases, BAT has a 10% share of the market and should thereby be held responsible for the deaths of 10,000 people each year.

Chris Proctor seems to be a kind of unofficial punch-bag for BAT. He's courteous and quiet-spoken and admits, more or less, to everything you care to throw at him: yes, it is a dilemma to be working for a tobacco company; yes, he would consider resigning if BAT wasn't striving to develop safer ways of putting the poison nicotine into your body. He believes if BAT ceased production of cigarettes tomorrow it would make no difference to public health, presumably because their customers would switch to other brands and they only have 10% of the UK market anyway. This I found unconvincing: BAT is one of the 'Big Four' tobacco companies, with 19% of the cigarette global market.[89] In any case, it's a very weak argument. If something is wrong in itself one shouldn't do it, even if someone else will. Examples that are often cited are atomic warfare research and the controller of the gas supply at Belsen.

To help BAT staff deal with the dilemma of working in such a company they have annual visits from an ethicist. When I heard this it made me feel sick. The identity of this ethicist, unsurprisingly, is confidential, but I couldn't help wondering whether it might be the philosopher Roger Scruton who has been paid by Japan Tobacco to promote sales of cigarettes[90] and who has criticised the WHO's campaign against smoking.[91]

What about Chris Proctor resigning from BAT? Not until the kids are off his hands – the 'I vos only trying to pay ze mortgage' excuse.

I am mildly curious what his kids think about his job. Are they proud their Daddy works for a tobacco company? Of

---

[89] BMJ 2015;350:h2052
[90] http://www.theguardian.com/media/2002/jan/24/advertising.tobaccoadvertising
[91] https://industrydocuments.library.ucsf.edu/tobacco/docs/#id=zpwk0052

course, it's not easy to admit that nearly three decades of your life's work have been a mistake. Nonetheless, if even now he turned his back on tobacco he might influence others in the industry to do the same. He could be a hero!

Unfortunately, there doesn't seem to be much chance of that happening.

Chapter 26

A Bulldog Named Gladys

She never lets up. Judge Gladys Kessler has got her teeth into the tobacco companies in America.

After finding in 2006 that several major tobacco companies had lied to the public about the harm which cigarettes cause, she is now trying to insist that they publish in a variety of media for specified periods, 'corrective statements' containing information of the following kind:

- Smoking kills on average 1,200 Americans every day
- More people die every year from smoking than from murder, AIDS, suicide, drugs, car crashes and alcohol combined
- Smoking causes heart disease, emphysema, acute myeloid leukemia, and cancer of the mouth, esophagus, larynx, lung, stomach, kidney, bladder and pancreas
- Smoking also causes reduced fertility, low birth weight in newborns and cancer of the cervix
- Smoking is highly addictive. Nicotine is the addictive drug in tobacco
- Cigarette companies intentionally designed cigarettes with enough nicotine to create and sustain addiction
- It's not easy to quit
- When you smoke, the nicotine actually changes the brain - that's why quitting is so hard
- Etc.

The tobacco companies are resisting this measure because, as they not unreasonably point out, they don't want to have to brand themselves as liars – even though they are. Now, apart from this, would the good Judge be so kind as to tell us what she is trying to achieve. Does she want to punish Big Tobacco, rather like a naughty school child being made to write out a hundred lines? Does she think she is telling the public stuff they don't know? (I would disagree with the statement that it's not easy to quit.) Is she trying to make people stop smoking through fear? One may speculate on all this but I think it misses the point.

What should happen, in my view, is that a lawsuit should be brought against the US *government* for knowingly allowing a product to be sold which:

- Kills on average 1,200 Americans every day – more than die every year from murder, AIDS, suicide, drugs, car crashes and alcohol, combined
- Causes heart disease, emphysema…etc.
- Is highly addictive
- Etc.

Further, I would seek to force the government to issue corrective statements that they failed in their duty to protect the public by leaving it up to the consciences of those decent people who run tobacco companies to put themselves out of business.

APPENDIX

The Symonds Method

In this appendix I explain how a simple understanding of the mechanism of nicotine addiction can enable smokers to quit easily and permanently. What follows is an outline; the full method is set out in my previous book, *Stop Smoking: Real Help at Last*.

I ask the patient, 'When you are at the point where you want the next cigarette, you feel something. But *what* do you feel?'

The immediate answer is usually 'I don't know' or 'Nothing' or 'I feel like I want a cigarette'. Well, what does it feel like to want a cigarette?

After back-and-forth questions and answers of this sort for a while, I may have to invent a scenario such as this: 'You're in a non-smoking meeting which goes on longer than expected and were looking forward to having a cigarette, but now have to put this off for another thirty minutes, what would you feel?' The reply may be, 'I don't know, I've never been in that situation!' Eventually the smoker will admit that he or she feels mildly anxious or stressed or nervous. The conversation, with my questions or comments in italics, then usually goes something like this:

Is there any physical pain?
No, of course not.

So you're feeling a bit nervous because you can't have a cigarette when you want one, and what will happen as time goes by?
It will get worse, I suppose.

And then what will happen?

I don't know, but I expect it will be very uncomfortable.

Would it ever become intolerable?
No, I don't think so.

So, if you still can't smoke, what will happen to the discomfort?
I suppose it will go away!

That's right: it will go away! And it will never come back – unless you put more nicotine into your body, which, of course, you will never want to do again.

Why do smokers feel nervous, anxious or uncomfortable when they haven't smoked for a while? The answer is as follows.

The smoker has got used to having a certain level of nicotine in his or her bloodstream and brain. Nicotine is a poison, and the body's excretory (cleansing) systems work overtime to get rid of it, mainly in the urine. When the nicotine has fallen to a certain level the smoker may begin to experience *withdrawal symptoms*. I say 'may' because for many smokers these symptoms are so mild they find it difficult to describe anything at all, or it may manifest itself only as vague uneasiness or a distracted feeling. These mildly uncomfortable withdrawal symptoms are interpreted, correctly, as a need for another cigarette. If you have one, these feeling are immediately relieved – but only until you want the next one!

It is essential for the smoker to understand that smoking is a self-perpetuating activity: each cigarette creates the need for the next one. Therefore, if you break the cycle by not putting anymore nicotine (in any form) into your body, these feelings will go away. There may be intermittent mild discomfort for a few days, but will it be unbearable? Only if you think it will! Instead, one can even enjoy these feelings by reminding oneself that *this is what it feels like as the nicotine is being cleansed for the last*

Smoking is a Psychological Problem

time from your body. You can then look forward to feeling well (other things being equal), free from anxiety and nervousness caused by nicotine withdrawal, for the rest of your life.

This is the Symonds Method in a nutshell. In practice, however, rather more explanation and support are often needed to change smokers' attitudes so that they have no wish to smoke ever again. After all, there should be no difficulty in refraining from something you don't want to do!

One of the main problems with the conventional approach to smoking cessation will be apparent if you look up nicotine withdrawal symptoms on the internet. (Google yielded 451,000 results.) You will find long lists of symptoms including headache, nausea, insomnia, constipation, irritability, anxiety, depression, difficulty in concentrating, increased appetite, tiredness and 'cravings'.

There is one serious objection to these lists of symptoms: *they are largely untrue.* Of the hundreds of smokers I have questioned face-to-face about what they actually feel when they are in a state of nicotine withdrawal, hardly anyone mentions most of these symptoms. As indicated above, typically all they say is that they feel mildly anxious or distracted. It is exceedingly rare for smokers to say they experience insomnia, nausea, depression, etc. One patient told me he suffered headaches when he didn't smoke, which was why he couldn't stop. I prescribed a painkiller for a few days.

Another patient, who I am sorry to say couldn't get beyond the stage of admitting to himself that he didn't really want to stop, told me every morning he felt such anxiety and depression that he was unable to concentrate on his work as a free-lance writer – a serious problem for him.

I suppose he could be put in the category of 'difficult' smokers, though the difficulty I think lay in his inability to recognize the real problem. This is a letter I sent him when I heard he hadn't stopped:

Dear Mr...

Let us summarize what has emerged so far.

For the first 24 hours after stopping all you are aware of is a mild mental discomfort. However, on waking the next morning you experience such anxiety and depression (AD) that you are unable to work unless you relieve these symptoms by taking more nicotine into your body.

These unpleasant feelings are due to nicotine withdrawal. This is clearly shown by the fact that on mornings when you are not trying to stop smoking you have thirty puffs first thing to gain relief, so you can then go about your normal activities.

You need these thirty puffs because you have not smoked during the night and your nicotine level on waking is at its lowest. Therefore, you are aware of the AD more strongly. Thereafter, during the day you only need ten puffs, repeated up to forty times (!), in order to keep the AD at bay so you can feel comfortable.

This means you must be dreading going to sleep each night, because you know the following morning you will wake up feeling overwhelmed by AD.

However, if you do not relieve the AD in the morning by another dose of nicotine (a large one contained in thirty inhalations of cigarette smoke), what will happen? The AD will go away!

I suspect there is an element of using the AD as an excuse, perhaps unconsciously, thus: 'I don't really want to stop smoking. I experience withdrawal symptoms when I awake in the mornings. Therefore I can't stop smoking.'

Taking you at your word that you do feel unpleasant AD, you are facing a choice:

a) continue smoking and suffer AD every morning for the rest of your life, or

b) put up with it – even endure it – for a few days and then never have it again!

Putting up with the AD for a short while can be made easier by keeping in mind that it is wonderful to be able to wake up each morning and feel well (other things being equal) without a dose of poison!

Good wishes,

Another difficult patient was a friend I used to have who was a smoker. Though intelligent and highly educated, he also didn't get it. I went through my method twice with him but he didn't stop, so I offered a third session. This he declined, saying 'I know your spiel.' However, he stopped a year later after he had a coronary artery by-pass operation.

END